# THE
# O POINT WEIGHT LOSS
# COOKBOOK

Easy Delicious Recipes, including Color Pictures, Health Benefits, Nutritional Value, 30-Days Meal Plan and more

# DR. ELAINE WAGONER

# TABLE OF CONTENTS

## LUNCH

Pineapple Chicken and Rice Wraps

Buffalo Chicken Wraps

White Chicken Chili Tacos

Broccoli Salad

Turkey Taco Pasta Salad

Turkey Burgers

BBQ Chicken Tostadas

Chicken Taco Cupcakes

Chicken Bacon Tostadas

## DINNER RECIPES

Salmon with Roasted Vegetables

Lentil Soup

Shrimp Scampi with Zoodles

Greek Chicken Salad

Black Bean Burgers

Chicken Taco Soup

Yogurt Chicken Salads and Dressings

Baked Salmon with Lemon and Dill

Yogurt Chicken Marinade

Buffalo Chicken Celery Bites

## SNACKS AND APPETIZERS RECIPES

Edamame

Air-Popped Popcorn

Hard-Boiled Eggs

Pickles

Soup Broth

Roasted Chickpeas

Cucumber Slices with Hummus

Apple Slices with Almond Butter

Celery Sticks with Cream Cheese

## DESSERTS RECIPES

Sugar-Free Jello Cups

Fruit Kabobs

Chia Seed Pudding

Cucumber Mint Sorbet

Rice Cake with Almond Butter

Stuffed Dates

Mixed Berry Smoothie

Banana "Ice Cream"

Greek Yogurt with Honey and Cinnamon

Watermelon Popsicles

# INTRODUCTION

Many of you have come to me on this health and wellness journey. You've indicated a wish to lose some weight, but the limitations of counting and measuring may have discouraged you. Here's some excellent news! This book provides a new road, one paved with tasty, fulfilling meals, all free of the weight of points.

*These pages include a plethora of dishes, each meticulously prepared to fuel your body while tantalizing your taste senses. We'll look at breakfasts to stimulate your mornings, lunches to keep you going all day, and dinners to bring your family together for a delicious and healthful experience.*

So, whether you're an experienced chef or just starting, this book welcomes you. Let us go on this adventure of discovery together, one delectable taste at a time.

# BREAKFAST
## Recipes

# FRESH FRUIT SALAD

## Ingredients

- 2 cups sliced strawberries
- 1 cup blueberries
- 1 cup diced cantaloupe
- 1/2 cup diced honeydew melon
- 1 kiwi, peeled and sliced
- 1 orange, segmented (or 1 cup mandarin oranges) 1/4 cup fresh mint leaves, chopped (optional)

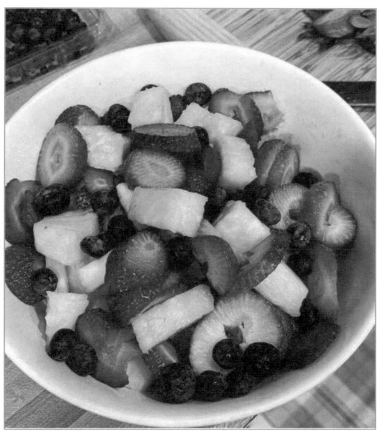

## Directions

- In a large bowl, gently combine all the fruits. If using mint, toss it in delicately to avoid bruising the leaves.

- (Optional) For a touch of zesty elegance, consider drizzling the fruit salad with a tablespoon of fresh lime or orange juice.

- Serve chilled and savor the explosion of flavors in each delightful bite.

 **Preparation Time : 10 min**

 **Total Time : 10 min**

 **Servings : 4**

 **Cooking Time: N/A**

## Nutritional Information

- Calories: 60
- Fat: 0g
- Saturated Fat: 0g
- Cholesterol: 0mg
- Sodium: 1mg
- Carbohydrates: 15g
- Fiber: 2g
- Sugars: 12g
- Protein: 1g

## Ingredients

- 1/2 cup rolled barley
- 1 cup unsweetened almond milk (or other zero-point plant-based milk)
- 1/4 cup mashed banana (about 1/2 banana)
- 1/2 teaspoon ground cinnamon
- 1/4 teaspoon baking powder
- 1/4 teaspoon salt
- 1 small apple, thinly sliced (about 1/2 cup)

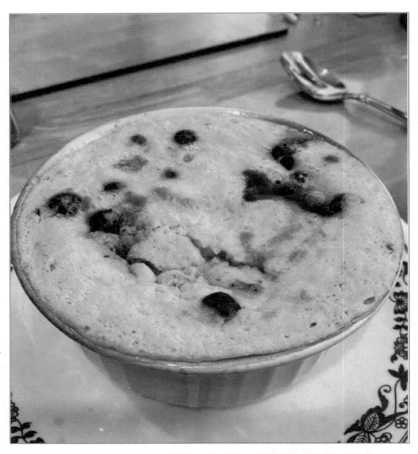

## Directions

1. In a medium bowl, combine the rolled barley and almond milk. Let sit for 5 minutes, allowing the barley to soften slightly.
2. Mash the banana in a separate bowl. Stir the mashed banana, cinnamon, baking powder, and salt into the barley mixture.
3. Fold in the sliced apples. Be gentle to avoid breaking the apple slices.
4. Heat a lightly greased non-stick pan over medium heat. Using a measuring cup or spoon, portion the batter evenly onto the pan.
5. Cook for 3-4 minutes per side, or until golden brown and cooked through. You may need to adjust the heat slightly to prevent burning.
6. Serve immediately and enjoy.

 **Preparation Time : 5 min**

 **Total Time : 20 min**

 **Servings : 2**

 **Cooking Time: 15 min**

## Nutritional Information

- Calories: 180
- Fat: 3g
- Carbohydrates: 32g
- Fiber: 5g
- Sugar: 8g
- Protein: 4g

# TOFU SCRAMBLED EGG

## Ingredients

- 4 ounces firm tofu, drained and crumbled
- 1/2 teaspoon minced
- garlic 1/4 cup chopped
- onion
  1 teaspoon nutritional
- yeast
- 1 teaspoon turmeric
- 2 teaspoons garlic powder
  Salt and freshly ground
- black pepper, to taste
  Cooking spray (zero-point option)

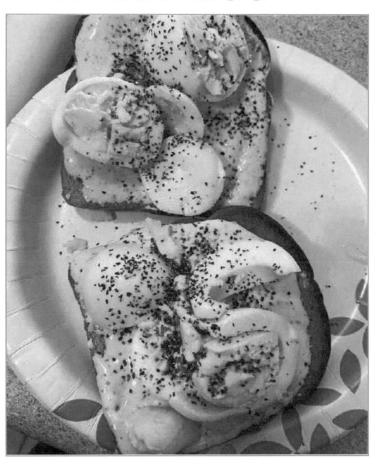

## Directions

1. In a small bowl, crumble the tofu with your hands, aiming for pieces resembling scrambled eggs. In a separate bowl, whisk together the nutritional yeast, turmeric, and garlic powder.

2. Heat a non-stick skillet over medium heat. Coat the pan with a light spray of cooking spray. Add the onions and saute until softened and translucent, about 3 minutes. Release the fragrant melody of the garlic by adding it for another minute, taking care not to burn it.

3. Increase the heat slightly. Add the crumbled tofu to the pan and cook for another 3-4 minutes, stirring frequently to prevent sticking.

4. Pour the nutritional yeast, turmeric, and garlic powder mixture over the tofu. Season generously with salt and pepper. Scramble everything together until well combined and heated through, about 2 minutes.

5. Plate your masterpiece and savor the deliciousness.

 **Preparation Time : 5 min**

 **Total Time : 15 min**

 **Servings : 1**

 **Cooking Time: 10 min**

## Nutritional Information

- Calories: 140
- Fat: 4g
- Carbohydrates: 5g
- Protein: 14g

## Ingredients

- 1 pound ground turkey breast (99% lean)
- 1 tablespoon ground sage
- 1 teaspoon dried thyme
- 1/2 teaspoon smoked paprika
- 1/4 teaspoon ground black pepper
- 1/4 teaspoon garlic powder
- 1/4 teaspoon onion powder
- Pinch of cayenne pepper (optional)
- Salt, to taste

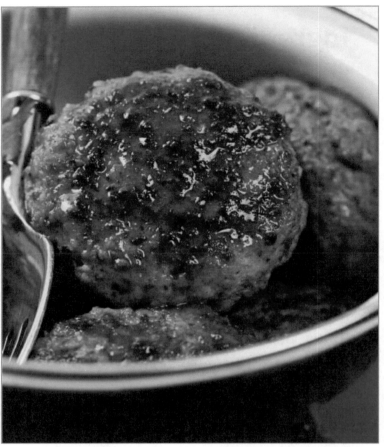

## Directions

1. In a large bowl, combine the ground turkey breast, sage, thyme, paprika, black pepper, garlic powder, onion powder, and cayenne pepper (if using). Using your hands, gently massage the spices into the meat until evenly distributed.
2. Portion the seasoned turkey mixture into 6 equal parts. Shape each portion into a compact patty, about 1/2-inch thick.
3. Heat a large nonstick skillet over medium heat. Spray the pan with a light coating of cooking spray. Gently add the patties to the skillet, leaving space between them.
4. Cook the patties for 5-7 minutes per side, or until browned and cooked through. A meat thermometer inserted into the center of a patty should register 165°F (74°C) for safe consumption.
5. Transfer the cooked patties to a plate lined with paper towels to drain any excess grease. Serve immediately and savor the deliciousness.

 **Preparation Time : 10 min**

 **Total Time : 25 min**

 **Servings : 6**

 **Cooking Time: 15 min**

## Nutritional Information

- Calories: 130
- Fat: 5g
- Carbs: 0g
- Protein: 18g

# SHAKSHUSKA

## Ingredients

- 1 tablespoon cooking spray
- 1 medium red onion, finely chopped
- 1 green bell pepper, finely chopped
- 2 cloves garlic, minced
- 1 teaspoon ground cumin
- 1/2 teaspoon smoked paprika
- 1 (14.5-ounce) can diced tomatoes, undrained
- 1/4 cup chopped fresh cilantro
- 4 large eggs
- Salt and freshly ground black pepper, to taste

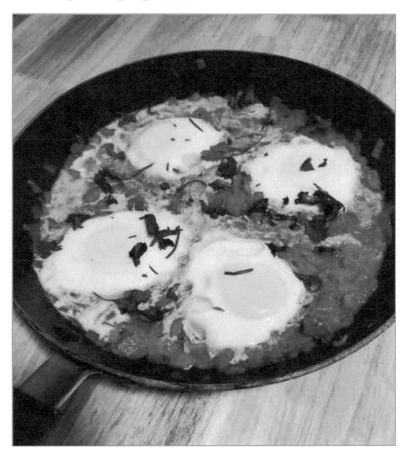

## Directions

1. In a large skillet, heat the cooking spray over medium heat. Sauté the onion and bell pepper until softened and translucent, about 5 minutes. Add the garlic, cumin, and paprika, and cook for an additional minute, allowing the spices to bloom.
2. Pour in the diced tomatoes and their juices, scraping up any browned bits from the bottom of the pan. Bring to a simmer, then reduce heat to low and let the sauce simmer for 10 minutes, allowing it to thicken slightly.
3. Using the back of a spoon, create four wells in the simmering sauce. Gently crack an egg into each well. Season with salt and pepper to taste.
4. Cover the skillet and simmer for 5-7 minutes, or until the egg whites are set and the yolks are cooked to your desired doneness.
5. Remove from heat and garnish with fresh cilantro.

 **Preparation Time : 5 min**

 **Total Time : 25 min**

 **Servings : 2**

 **Cooking Time: 20 min**

## Nutritional Information

- Calories: 210
- Fat: 7g
- Carbohydrates: 17g
- Fiber: 3g
- Protein: 12g

## Ingredients

- 12 large eggs
- 1/4 cup chopped vegetables (such as bell pepper, onion, spinach, or mushrooms) - optional
- 1/4 cup shredded reduced-fat cheese - optional
- 1/4 teaspoon dried herbs (such as oregano, basil, or thyme) - optional
- Salt and freshly ground black pepper, to taste
- Cooking spray

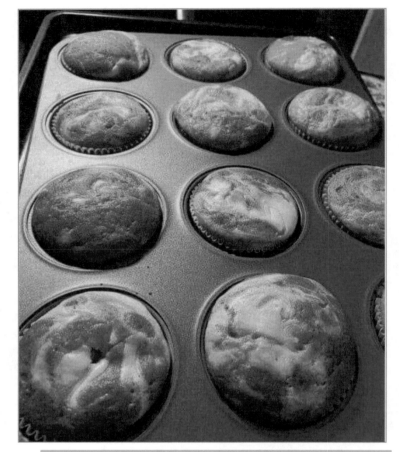

## Directions

1. Preheat your oven to 375°F (190°C). Lightly grease a 12-cup muffin tin with cooking spray.
2. In a large bowl, whisk together the eggs. If using, gently fold in your chosen vegetables, cheese, and herbs. Season generously with salt and pepper.
3. Divide the egg mixture evenly among the prepared muffin cups.
4. Bake for 15-20 minutes, or until the eggs are set and the centers are no longer runny. A toothpick inserted into the center should come out clean.
5. Let cool slightly before removing from the muffin tin. Serve warm or store in an airtight container in the refrigerator for up to 3 days.

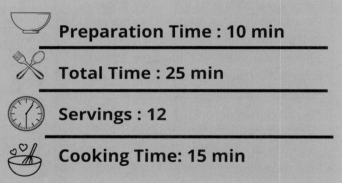

**Preparation Time : 10 min**

**Total Time : 25 min**

**Servings : 12**

**Cooking Time: 15 min**

## Nutritional Information

- Calories: 70
- Fat: 5g
- Carbohydrates: 1g
- Protein: 6g

# BANANA BERRY PARFAIT

## Ingredients

- 1/2 cup non-fat Greek yogurt
- 1/2 banana, sliced
- 1/2 cup mixed
- berries 1/4 teaspoon ground cinnamon
- Optional: A sprig of mint for garnish

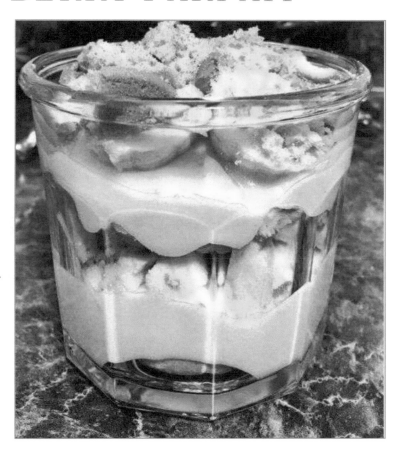

## Directions

1. In a beautiful glass (because presentation matters!), layer half of the non-fat Greek yogurt.
2. Scatter half of the sliced banana on top of the yogurt, creating a mosaic of sunshine yellow.
3. Next, add a vibrant layer of half the mixed berries. Imagine them as jewels adorning your culinary creation.
4. Repeat steps 1-3 to create another layer of yogurt, banana, and berries.
5. Sprinkle the ground cinnamon over the top, like a dusting of fragrant snow.

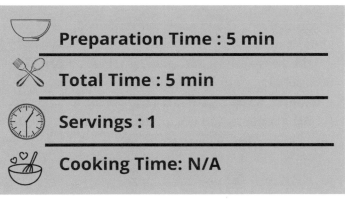

Preparation Time : 5 min

Total Time : 5 min

Servings : 1

Cooking Time: N/A

## Nutritional Information

- Calories: 130 | Fat: 0g
- Saturated Fat: 0g | Cholesterol: 5mg
- Sodium: 35mg | Carbohydrates: 21g
- Fiber: 3g | Sugar: 15g
- Protein: 10g

## Ingredients

- 1 bunch silverbeet, roughly chopped
- 1 tablespoon olive oil
- 1/2 small onion, diced
- 1 clove garlic, minced (optional)
- 1 small tomato, diced (optional)
- Salt and freshly ground black pepper, to taste
- 2 large eggs
- 1/4 cup crumbled feta cheese
- 2 tablespoons dukkah

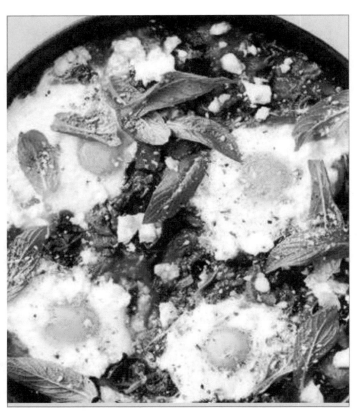

## Directions

1. Preheat your oven to 180°C (350°F) or 160°C (320°F) fan-forced.
2. In a large saucepan, heat olive oil over medium heat. Add the onion (and garlic, if using) and cook until softened, about 5 minutes.
3. Add the silverbeet and cook, stirring occasionally, until wilted, about 2 minutes. Season with salt and pepper. (If using tomato, add it with the silverbeet and cook until softened)
4. Divide the silverbeet mixture between two oven-safe ramekins or small baking dishes. Create a shallow well in the center of each portion.
5. Crack an egg into each well. Season with a pinch of salt and pepper.
6. Sprinkle the feta cheese and dukkah over each egg.
7. Bake for 10-12 minutes, or until the egg whites are set and the yolks are cooked to your desired doneness.
8. pen_spark

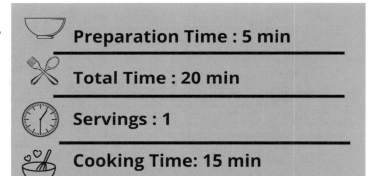

**Preparation Time : 5 min**

**Total Time : 20 min**

**Servings : 1**

**Cooking Time: 15 min**

## Nutritional Information

- Calories: 230
- Fat: 12g
- Carbs: 10g
- Protein: 15g

# POACHED EGGS AND TOAST

## Ingredients

- 1 large, free-range egg (room temperature)
- 1 slice whole-wheat bread
- Freshly ground black pepper, to taste
- Optional: Chopped fresh chives or parsley, for garnish

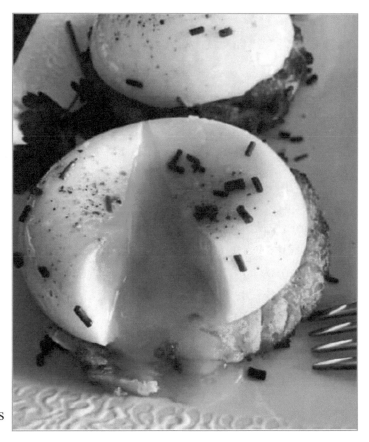

## Directions

1. Fill a small saucepan with 2 inches of water and bring to a simmer.
2. While the water heats, toast your bread to your desired level of crispness.
3. Crack the egg into a small bowl. Using a spoon, gently swirl the water to create a vortex. Slowly pour the egg into the center of the vortex.
4. Cook for 3-4 minutes, or until the whites are set but the yolk is still runny.
5. Using a slotted spoon, carefully lift the poached egg from the water and place it on top of the toast.
6. Season with freshly ground black pepper and garnish with chopped chives or parsley, if desired.

 **Preparation Time : 5 min**

 **Total Time : 20 min**

 **Servings : 1**

 **Cooking Time: 10 min**

## Nutritional Information

- Calories: 190
- Protein:  12g
- Fat: 9g
- Carbs: 14g
- Fiber: 2g

## Ingredients

- 6 slices center-cut bacon, chopped
- 10 ounces fresh baby spinach
- 6 large eggs
- 1/2 cup shredded part-skim mozzarella cheese
- 1/4 teaspoon dried oregano
- Salt and freshly ground black pepper, to taste

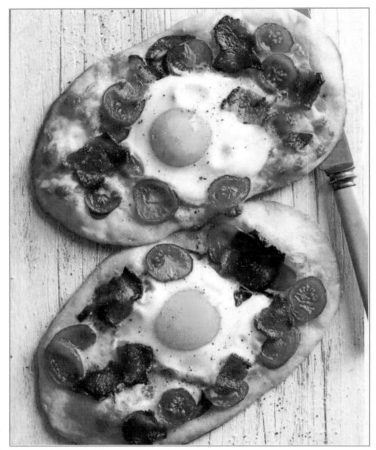

## Directions

1. Preheat oven to 375°F (190°C). Lightly grease a six-cup muffin tin.
2. In a large skillet over medium heat, cook bacon until crisp. Remove with a slotted spoon and drain on paper towels.
3. Wilt spinach in the bacon drippings until softened. Drain any excess liquid.
4. In a large bowl, whisk together eggs, cheese, oregano, salt, and pepper.
5. Divide the spinach and bacon evenly among the muffin cups. Pour egg mixture over top.
6. Bake for 20-22 minutes, or until the eggs are set and the tops are golden brown.

 **Preparation Time : 5 min**

 **Total Time : 25 min**

 **Servings : 6**

 **Cooking Time: 20 min**

## Nutritional Information

- Calories: 140
- Fat: 8g
- Carbohydrates : 2g
- Protein: 12g

## Ingredients

- 1 large, fresh egg
- 1 large, ripe tomato, diced
- 1/4 red onion, finely chopped
- 1 tablespoon chopped fresh cilantro
- 1 tablespoon fresh lime juice
- Pinch of chili powder (optional)
- Salt and freshly ground black pepper, to taste

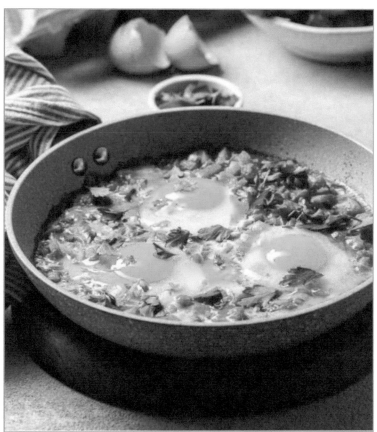

## Directions

1. In a small bowl, combine diced tomato, red onion, cilantro, lime juice, chili powder (if using), salt, and pepper. Stir gently to combine.
2. Fill a shallow pan with about 2 inches of water. Bring to a simmer over medium heat. Crack the egg into a small bowl.
3. Once the water simmers, create a gentle vortex by swirling the water with a spoon. Carefully slide the egg into the center of the vortex. Cook for 3-4 minutes for a runny yolk, or adjust time for desired doneness.
4. While the egg poaches, prepare your toast or a bed of greens (optional) for serving.
5. Using a slotted spoon, gently transfer the poached egg to your serving plate. Spoon the vibrant tomato salsa around the egg.

 **Preparation Time : 5 min**

 **Total Time : 15 min**

 **Servings : 1**

 **Cooking Time: 10 min**

## Nutritional Information

- Calories: 170
- Fat: 5g
- Carbohydrates : 12g
- Protein: 12g

## Ingredients

- 1/2 peach, pitted and halved
- 1/2 pineapple ring, cored
- 1/4 cup fresh raspberries
- 1/4 cup blueberries
- 1 sprig fresh mint, for garnish (optional)

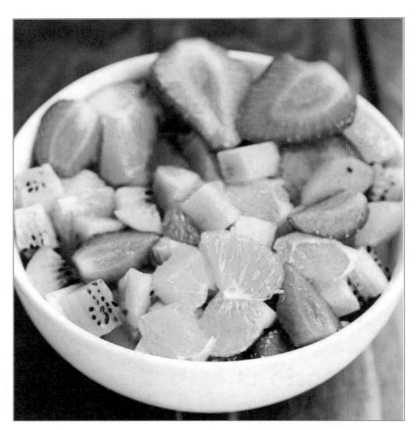

## Directions

1. Preheat a grill pan or grill to medium-high heat.
2. Brush the cut sides of the peach and pineapple with a touch of water to prevent sticking. Grill each piece for 2-3 minutes per side, or until lightly charred and softened.
3. In a bowl, combine the grilled fruit, raspberries, and blueberries. Toss gently.

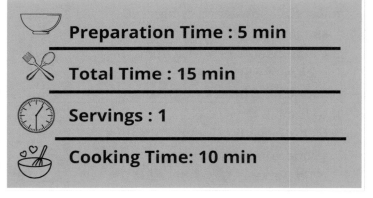

**Preparation Time : 5 min**

**Total Time : 15 min**

**Servings : 1**

**Cooking Time: 10 min**

## Nutritional Information

- Calories: 60
- Fat: 0g
- Carbohydrates: 15g
- Fiber: 3g
- Sugar: 10g

## Ingredients

- 2 medium sweet potatoes, peeled and diced
- 1 red bell pepper, diced
- 1/2 red onion, diced
- 2 cloves garlic, minced
- 1 tablespoon olive oil
- 1 teaspoon dried thyme
- 1/2 teaspoon smoked paprika
- Salt and freshly ground black pepper, to taste

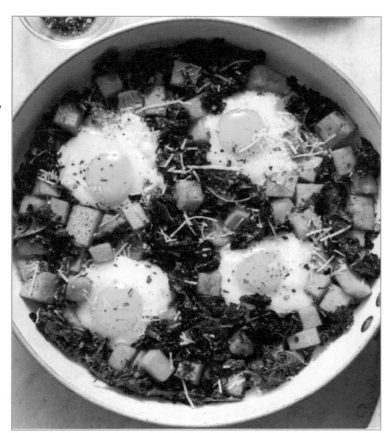

## Directions

1. Preheat oven to 425°F (220°C). Line a baking sheet with parchment paper.
2. In a large bowl, toss sweet potatoes, bell pepper, red onion, olive oil, thyme, paprika, salt, and pepper. Spread evenly on the prepared baking sheet.
3. Roast for 30 minutes, or until vegetables are tender and golden brown, flipping halfway through.
4. Remove from oven and serve immediately.

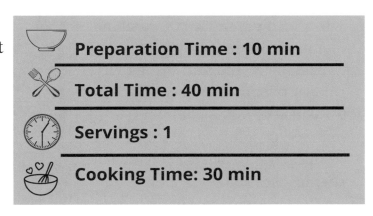

**Preparation Time : 10 min**

**Total Time : 40 min**

**Servings : 1**

**Cooking Time: 30 min**

## Nutritional Information

- Calories: 180
- Carbohydrates: 30g
- Fiber: 5g
- Sugar: 8g
- Fat: 3g

# STRAWBERRY OATMEAL

## Ingredients

- 1 cup rolled oats (old-fashioned or quick)
- 1 ¾ cups unsweetened almond milk (or low-fat milk of choice)
- ¾ cup water
- ½ pound fresh strawberries, hulled and sliced
- 1 tablespoon granulated sugar (optional)
- ½ teaspoon vanilla extract
- ¼ teaspoon ground cinnamon
- Pinch of salt

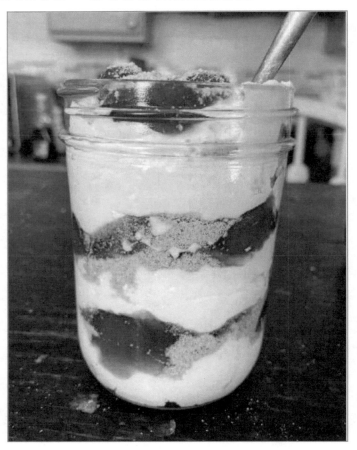

## Directions

1. In a medium saucepan, combine almond milk, water, oats, cinnamon, and salt. Bring to a simmer over medium heat.
2. Reduce heat and cook for 5 minutes, or until oats are thickened to desired consistency, stirring occasionally.
3. While the oatmeal simmers, toss the strawberries with the sugar (if using) in a small bowl.
4. Remove the oatmeal from the heat and stir in the vanilla extract.
5. Spoon the oatmeal into a serving bowl and top generously with the sweet strawberry mixture.

 **Preparation Time : 5 min**

 **Total Time : 15 min**

 **Servings : 1**

 **Cooking Time: 10 min**

## Nutritional Information

- Calories: 230
- Fat: 3g
- Saturated Fat: 0.5g
- Carbohydrates: 40g
- Fiber: 4g
- Sugar: 5g (including natural sugars from strawberries)
- Protein: 5g

# BERRY BAKED OATS

## Ingredients

- ½ cup rolled oats (old-fashioned or quick-cooking)
- 1 ripe banana, mashed
- 1 large egg, beaten
- 1 teaspoon ground cinnamon
- ¼ teaspoon vanilla extract
- ½ cup unsweetened almond milk (or any zero-point milk)
- ½ cup mixed berries (fresh or frozen)

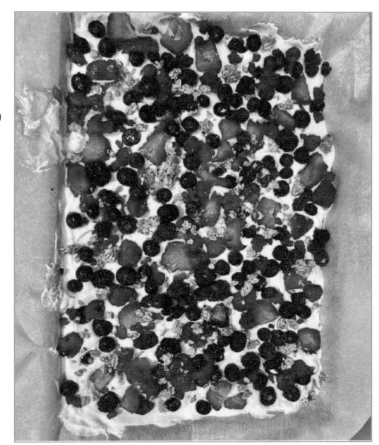

## Directions

1. Preheat your oven to 350°F (175°C). Lightly grease a single ramekin.
2. In a bowl, whisk together the oats, mashed banana, egg, cinnamon, and vanilla extract.
3. Stir in the almond milk and gently fold in the berries.
4. Pour the batter into the prepared ramekin and bake for 20-22 minutes, or until a toothpick inserted into the center comes out clean.

 **Preparation Time : 5 min**

 **Total Time : 25 min**

 **Servings : 1**

 **Cooking Time: 20 min**

## Nutritional Information

- Calories: 230
- Fat: 3g
- Carbohydrates: 40g
- Fiber: 4g
- Sugar: 12g
- Protein: 6g

# LUNCH

Recipes

## Ingredients

- 1 tablespoon olive oil
- 1 pound boneless, skinless chicken breasts, cubed
- 1/2 cup chopped fresh pineapple
- 1/4 cup low-sodium soy sauce
- 2 tablespoons brown sugar substitute
- 1 tablespoon cornstarch
- 1 cup cooked brown rice
- 4 whole wheat wraps
- Cilantro, chopped (for garnish)
- Red bell pepper, thinly sliced (optional)

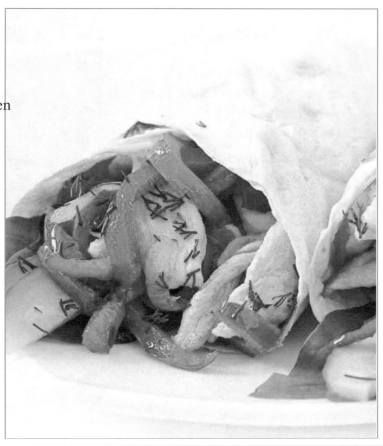

## Directions

1. Heat olive oil in a large skillet over medium heat. Add chicken and cook until golden brown and cooked through, about 8 minutes.
2. Stir in pineapple, soy sauce, and brown sugar substitute. Bring to a simmer and cook for 2 minutes.
3. In a small bowl, whisk together cornstarch and 1 tablespoon of water. Add to the pan and cook until the sauce thickens, about 1 minute.
4. Stir in cooked brown rice and heat through.
5. Spread chicken mixture evenly over each wrap. Garnish with cilantro and red bell pepper (optional).

 **Preparation Time : 10 min**

 **Total Time : 25 min**

 **Servings : 4**

 **Cooking Time: 15 min**

## Nutritional Information

- Calories: 350
- Fat: 7g
- Carbohydrates: 45g
- Fiber: 4g
- Protein: 25g

## Ingredients

- 1 pound boneless, skinless chicken breasts (poached, grilled, or baked)
- 1/4 cup Franks RedHot Original Wings & Things Hot Sauce (or your favorite zero-point hot sauce)
- 1 tablespoon light blue cheese dressing (or plain nonfat Greek yogurt)
- 2 large whole wheat tortillas (toasted, optional)
- Romaine lettuce, chopped
- Celery sticks, sliced (optional)
- Carrot sticks, sliced (optional)

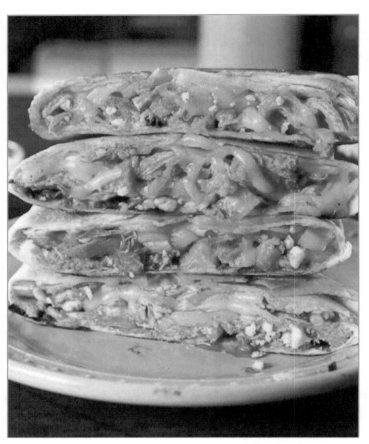

## Directions

1. Shred or chop the cooked chicken breasts.
2. In a bowl, toss the chicken with the hot sauce and blue cheese dressing (or yogurt) until evenly coated.
3. Spread the mixture onto the tortillas.
4. Top with lettuce, celery, and carrots (if using).
5. Roll up tightly and enjoy.

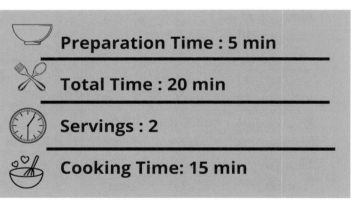

**Preparation Time : 5 min**

**Total Time : 20 min**

**Servings : 2**

**Cooking Time: 15 min**

## Nutritional Information

- Calories: 250
- Protein: 30g
- Carbs: 15g
- Fat: 5g

## Ingredients

- 14 small corn tortillas
- 1 ½ tablespoons unsalted butter
- 1 tablespoon all-purpose flour
- ½ cup skim milk
- ½ cup chicken broth
- 1 tablespoon chopped canned green chilies
- ¼ teaspoon cumin
- ¼ teaspoon chili powder
- Salt and pepper to taste
- 8 ounces shredded cooked chicken
- ¾ cup frozen corn
- ¼ cup chopped green onion
- 3.5 ounces shredded reduced-fat mozzarella cheese

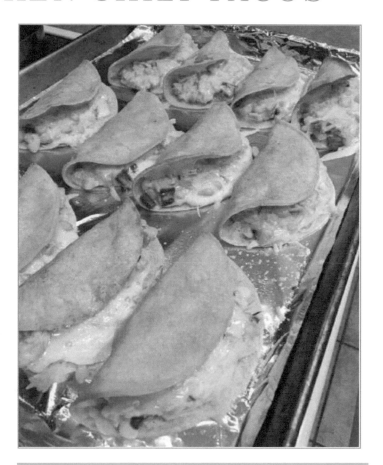

## Directions

1. In a skillet over medium heat, melt butter. Whisk in flour and cook for 1 minute. Slowly whisk in milk and broth, then bring to a simmer. Stir in green chilies, cumin, chili powder, salt, and pepper.
2. Reduce heat and simmer for 5 minutes. Add chicken and corn, and heat through.
3. Warm tortillas according to package directions.
4. Divide chicken chili mixture among tortillas. Top with green onion and cheese. Serve immediately.

 **Preparation Time : 10 min**

 **Total Time : 30 min**

 **Servings : 4**

 **Cooking Time: 20 min**

## Nutritional Information

- Calories: 300
- Fat: 7g
- Carbohydrates: 35g
- Fiber: 3g
- Protein: 25g

# BROCCOLI SALAD

## Ingredients

- 3 cups chopped broccoli florets
- 1/2 cup chopped red onion
- 1/4 cup chopped celery (optional, for extra crunch)
- 1/4 cup dried cranberries
- 1/4 cup chopped fresh dill or parsley

## Dressing

- 2 tablespoons fat-free Greek yogurt
- 1 tablespoon lemon juice
- 1 tablespoon Dijon mustard
- 1/4 teaspoon garlic powder
- Salt and freshly ground black pepper to taste

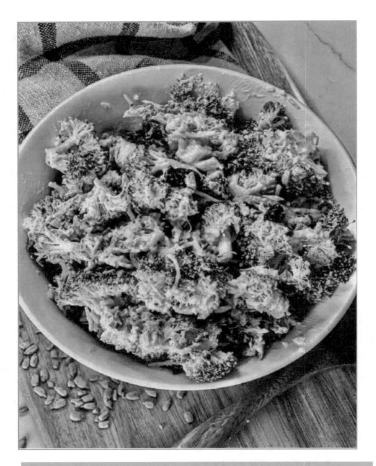

## Directions

1. In a large bowl, combine broccoli florets, red onion, celery (if using), and cranberries.
2. In a separate bowl, whisk together Greek yogurt, lemon juice, Dijon mustard, garlic powder, salt, and pepper.
3. Pour the dressing over the broccoli mixture and toss gently to combine.
4. Garnish with fresh dill or parsley before serving.

 **Preparation Time : 10 min**

 **Total Time : 10 min**

 **Servings : 4**

 **Cooking Time: N/A**

## Nutritional Information

- Calories: 50
- Fat: 0g
- Carbohydrates: 8g
- Fiber: 2g
- Sugar: 4g
- Protein: 2g

# TURKEY TACO PASTA SALAD

## Ingredients

- 1 pound ground turkey (93% lean or higher)
- 2.5 tablespoons taco seasoning
- 8 ounces whole-wheat rotini pasta (cooked according to package directions)
- 1 cup chopped bell peppers (any color)
- ½ cup diced red onion
- 1 cup grape tomatoes, halved
- 2 cups shredded romaine lettuce
- ½ cup fat-free shredded cheddar cheese
- ¼ cup light vinaigrette dressing (such as Italian or Catalina)

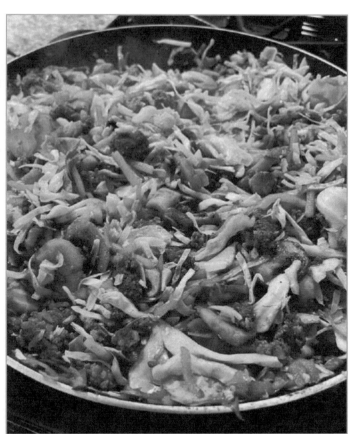

## Directions

1. In a large skillet, brown the ground turkey over medium heat, crumbling it as it cooks. Drain any excess fat.
2. Stir in the taco seasoning and cook for an additional minute, allowing the flavors to meld.
3. In a large bowl, combine the cooked pasta, cooled ground turkey mixture, bell peppers, red onion, and grape tomatoes.
4. Toss with the light vinaigrette dressing and gently fold in the shredded romaine lettuce.
5. Top with the fat-free cheddar cheese just before serving.

 **Preparation Time : 10 min**

 **Total Time : 25 min**

 **Servings : 4**

 **Cooking Time: 15 min**

## Nutritional Information

- Calories: 350
- Fat: 10g
- Carbohydrates: 40g
- Protein: 25g

# TURKEY BURGERS

## Ingredients

- 1 pound ground turkey breast (93% lean or higher)
- 1/2 cup finely chopped red onion
- 1/4 cup chopped fresh parsley
- 2 tablespoons Worcestershire sauce
- 1 tablespoon Dijon mustard
- 1 teaspoon dried thyme
- 1/2 teaspoon garlic powder
- Salt and freshly ground black pepper, to taste

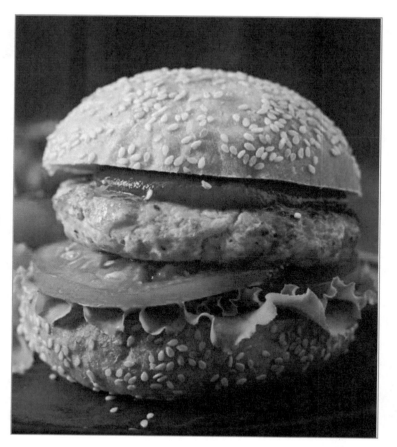

## Directions

1. In a large bowl, combine all ingredients gently but thoroughly.
2. Form the mixture into 4 equal patties.
3. Heat a grill pan or skillet over medium heat. Cook the burgers for 5-7 minutes per side, or until cooked through.

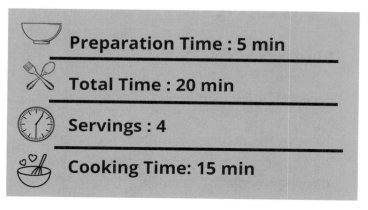

Preparation Time : 5 min

Total Time : 20 min

Servings : 4

Cooking Time: 15 min

## Nutritional Information

- Calories: 240
- Fat: 7g
- Carbohydrates: 2g
- Protein: 38g

# BBQ CHICKEN TOSTADAS

## Ingredients

- 2 corn tortillas
- 1 boneless, skinless chicken breast (cooked and shredded)
- 1/2 cup your favorite zero-point BBQ sauce
- 1/4 cup fat-free, shredded cheddar cheese
- 1/4 cup chopped red onion
- 1/4 cup chopped cilantro
- Lime wedges, for serving (optional)

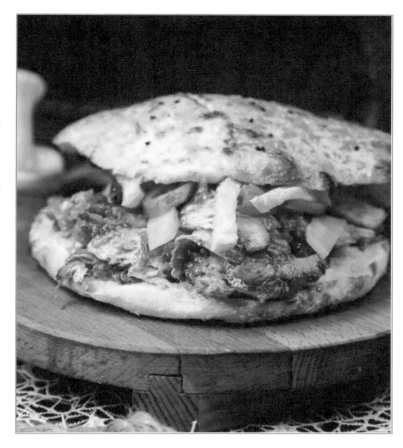

## Directions

1. Preheat oven to 400°F (200°C). Arrange tortillas on a baking sheet and bake for 5 minutes, or until crisp.
2. In a bowl, toss shredded chicken with BBQ sauce until evenly coated.
3. Divide the chicken mixture between the tortillas. Top with cheese, red onion, and cilantro.
4. Bake for an additional 5-7 minutes, or until cheese is melted and bubbly.

 **Preparation Time : 5 min**

 **Total Time : 20 min**

 **Servings : 2**

 **Cooking Time: 15 min**

## Nutritional Information

- Calories: 280
- Fat: 5g
- Carbohydrates: 30g
- Fiber: 3g
- Protein: 25g

# CHICKEN TACO CUPCAKES

## Ingredients

- 1 pound boneless, skinless chicken breasts, cooked and shredded
- 1 cup chopped tomatoes
- ½ cup chopped red onion
- 1 (15-ounce) can black beans, rinsed and drained
- 2 tablespoons taco seasoning
- ¼ cup chopped fresh cilantro
- 24 mini whole wheat tortillas

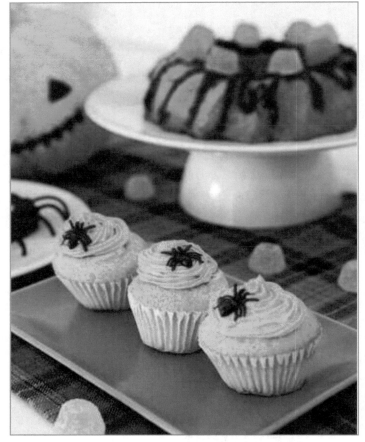

## Directions

1. In a large bowl, combine shredded chicken, tomatoes, red onion, black beans, taco seasoning, and cilantro. Toss gently to coat.
2. Preheat oven to 375°F (190°C). Lightly grease a mini muffin tin.
3. Press two mini tortillas into each greased muffin cup, forming a little cup shape. Fill each cup with the chicken mixture.
4. Bake for 15 minutes, or until tortillas are golden brown and filling is heated through.

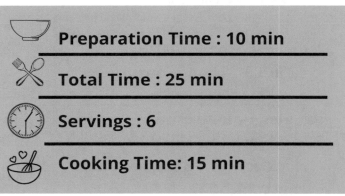

Preparation Time : 10 min

Total Time : 25 min

Servings : 6

Cooking Time: 15 min

## Nutritional Information

- Calories: 200
- Fat: 5g
- Carbohydrates: 25g
- Fiber: 5g
- Protein: 20g

# CHICKEN BACON TOSTADAS

## Ingredients

- 2 large round tostada shells
- 2 boneless, skinless chicken breasts, cooked and shredded
- 4 slices center-cut bacon, crisped and crumbled
- 1/2 cup chopped romaine lettuce
- 1/2 avocado, sliced
- 1/4 cup salsa fresca
- Chopped fresh cilantro, for garnish

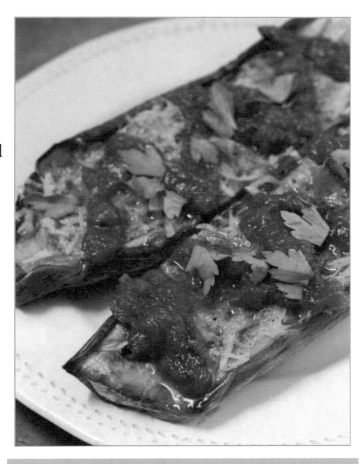

## Directions

1. Arrange the tostada shells on a serving platter.
2. Divide the shredded chicken and crumbled bacon evenly between the shells.
3. Top with romaine lettuce, avocado slices, and salsa fresca.
4. Garnish with fresh cilantro, and serve immediately.

 **Preparation Time : 10 min**

 **Total Time : 25 min**

 **Servings : 2**

 **Cooking Time: 15 min**

## Nutritional Information

- Calories: 350
- Fat: 15g
- Carbohydrates: 20g
- Fiber: 5g
- Protein: 30g

# DINNER
## Recipes

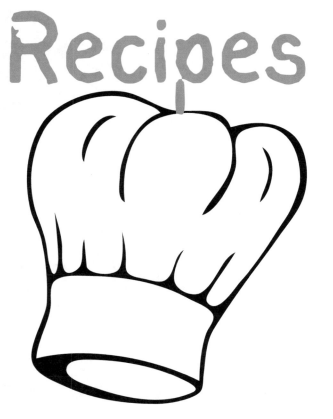

# SALMON WITH ROASTED VEGETABLES

## Ingredients

- 1 pound salmon fillets (skin-on or skinless, your preference)
- 1 medium zucchini, sliced into half-moons
- 1 medium red bell pepper, sliced into strips
- 1 medium yellow bell pepper, sliced into strips
- 1 red onion, thinly sliced
- 2 tablespoons olive oil
- 1 teaspoon dried oregano
- 1/2 teaspoon garlic powder
- Salt and freshly ground black pepper, to taste

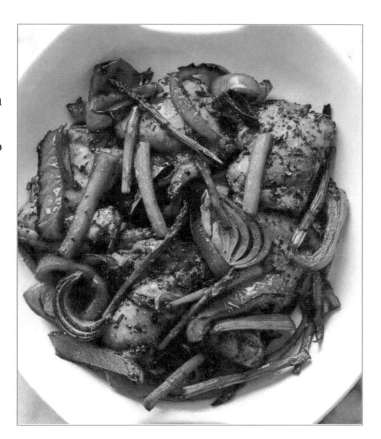

## Directions

1. Preheat oven to 425°F (220°C). Line a baking sheet with parchment paper.
2. In a large bowl, toss together zucchini, bell peppers, onion, olive oil, oregano, garlic powder, salt, and pepper. Spread the vegetables evenly on the prepared baking sheet.
3. Place the salmon fillets on top of the vegetables. Season the salmon with salt and pepper.
4. Roast for 20-25 minutes, or until the salmon is cooked through and flakes easily with a fork, and the vegetables are tender-crisp.

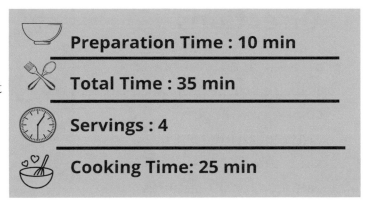

Preparation Time : 10 min

Total Time : 35 min

Servings : 4

Cooking Time: 25 min

## Nutritional Information

- Calories: 300
- Fat: 15g
- Carbohydrates: 10g
- Protein: 30g

## Ingredients

- 1 cup dried brown lentils, rinsed
- 4 cups low-sodium vegetable broth
- 2 carrots, chopped
- 2 celery stalks, chopped
- 1 onion, chopped
- 3 cloves garlic, minced
- 1 teaspoon dried thyme
- Salt and freshly ground black pepper, to taste
- Chopped fresh parsley, for garnish (optional)

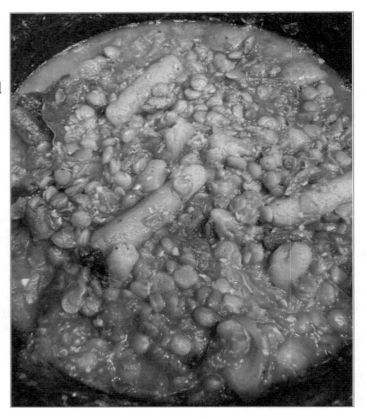

## Directions

1. In a large pot, combine lentils, broth, carrots, celery, onion, garlic, and thyme. Bring to a boil, then reduce heat and simmer for 30 minutes, or until lentils are tender.

2. Season with salt and pepper to taste. Ladle into bowls and garnish with fresh parsley, if desired.

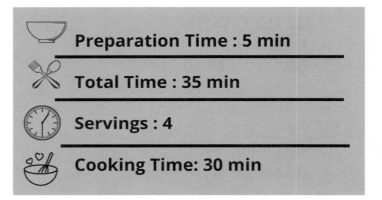

Preparation Time : 5 min

Total Time : 35 min

Servings : 4

Cooking Time: 30 min

## Nutritional Information

- Calories: 200
- Fat: 3g
- Carbohydrates: 30g
- Fiber: 8g
- Protein: 12g

## Ingredients

- 1 medium zucchini, spiralized into noodles (zoodles)
- 1 tablespoon olive oil
- 2 cloves garlic, minced
- 1/4 teaspoon red pepper flakes (optional)
- 1/2 pound large shrimp, peeled and deveined
- 2 tablespoons dry white wine or chicken broth
- 1 tablespoon fresh lemon juice
- 1/4 cup chopped fresh parsley
- Salt and freshly ground black pepper, to taste

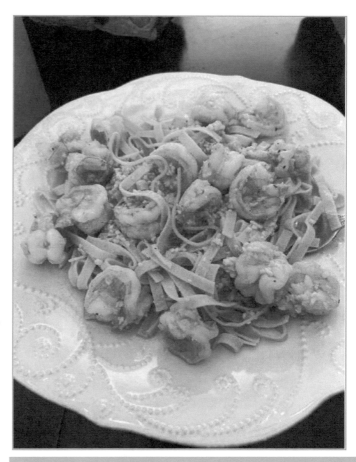

## Directions

1. In a large skillet, heat olive oil over medium heat. Add garlic and red pepper flakes (if using) and cook for 30 seconds, until fragrant.
2. Increase heat to medium-high and add shrimp. Season with salt and pepper. Cook for 2-3 minutes per side, or until pink and opaque.
3. Add white wine or broth and lemon juice to the pan, scraping up any browned bits. Simmer for 1 minute, allowing the sauce to reduce slightly.
4. Toss in zoodles and cook for 1-2 minutes, until heated through.
5. Remove from heat and stir in parsley. Season with additional salt and pepper, to taste.

 **Preparation Time : 5 min**

 **Total Time : 15 min**

 **Servings : 1**

 **Cooking Time: 10 min**

## Nutritional Information

- Calories: 200
- Fat: 7g
- Carbohydrates: 10g
- Fiber: 2g
- Protein: 20g

# GREEK CHICKEN SALAD

## Ingredients

- 2 cups cooked, shredded chicken breast (skinless, boneless)
- 1/2 cup chopped cucumber
- 1/4 cup crumbled feta cheese
- 1/4 cup chopped red onion
- 1/4 cup chopped kalamata olives
- 2 tablespoons chopped fresh dill
- 1 tablespoon fresh lemon juice
- 1 tablespoon olive oil
- 1/2 teaspoon dried oregano
- Salt and freshly ground black pepper, to taste

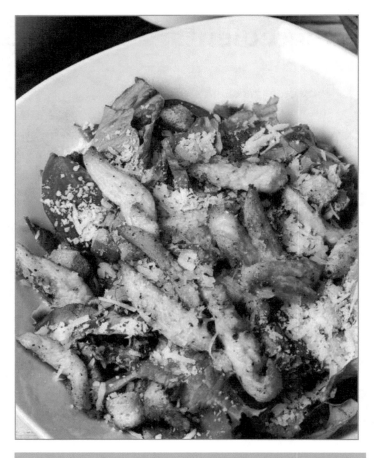

## Directions

1. In a large bowl, combine the shredded chicken, cucumber, feta cheese, red onion, olives, and dill.
2. In a small bowl, whisk together the lemon juice, olive oil, and oregano. Season with salt and pepper to taste.
3. Pour the dressing over the chicken salad and toss gently to coat.

 **Preparation Time : 10 min**

 **Total Time : 10 min**

 **Servings : 2**

 **Cooking Time:**

## Nutritional Information

- Calories: 240
- Fat: 8g
- Carbohydrates: 5g
- Fiber: 1g
- Protein: 32g

# BLACK BEAN BURGERS

## Ingredients

- 1 (15 oz) can black beans, rinsed and drained
- 1 cup cooked brown rice
- ½ red onion, finely chopped
- ½ green bell pepper, finely chopped
- 1 clove garlic, minced
- 1 jalapeño pepper, seeded and minced (optional)
- 1 tablespoon chopped fresh cilantro
- 1 teaspoon ground cumin
- ½ teaspoon chili powder
- ¼ teaspoon smoked paprika
- Salt and freshly ground black pepper, to taste
- Cooking spray

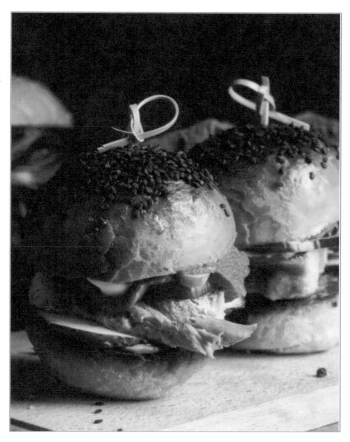

## Directions

1. In a large bowl, mash the black beans with a fork, leaving some texture. Add the cooked brown rice, red onion, bell pepper, garlic, jalapeño (if using), cilantro, cumin, chili powder, paprika, salt, and pepper. Stir until well combined.
2. Form the mixture into four equal patties. Lightly coat a skillet with cooking spray and heat over medium heat. Add the patties and cook for 5-7 minutes per side, or until golden brown and heated through.
3. Serve on whole-wheat buns with your favorite burger toppings.

 **Preparation Time : 10 min**

 **Total Time : 25 min**

 **Servings : 4**

 **Cooking Time: 15 min**

## Nutritional Information

- Calories: 250
- Fat: 5g
- Carbohydrates: 35g
- Fiber: 7g
- Protein: 15g

# CHICKEN TACO SOUP

## Ingredients

- 1 pound boneless, skinless chicken breasts
- 1 onion, chopped
- 2 garlic cloves, minced
- 1 (14.5 oz) can diced tomatoes, undrained
- 1 (15 oz) can tomato sauce
- 1 (15 oz) can black beans, rinsed and drained
- 1 (15 oz) can pinto beans, rinsed and drained
- 1 (15.25 oz) can corn, drained
- 4 cups chicken broth
- 1 ounce taco seasoning

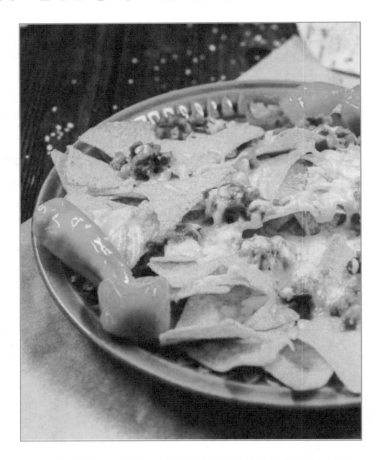

## Directions

1. In a large bowl, combine chicken, onion, garlic, diced tomatoes, tomato sauce, beans, corn, chicken broth, and taco seasoning. Stir well to coat.
2. Transfer mixture to your slow cooker and cook on low for 4 hours.
3. When ready to serve, shred the chicken directly in the slow cooker with two forks.

 **Preparation Time : 10 min**

 **Total Time : 4hrs 10 min**

 **Servings : 6**

 **Cooking Time: 4 hrs**

## Nutritional Information

- Calories: 230
- Fat: 3g
- Carbohydrates: 28g
- Fiber: 8g
- Protein: 25g

## Ingredients

- 2 cups cooked, shredded chicken breast (poached, grilled, or baked)
- 1 cup red grapes, halved
- 2 stalks celery, thinly sliced
- 1/4 cup chopped red onion (optional)
- 1/4 cup fat-free plain Greek yogurt
- 1 tablespoon lemon juice
- 1 tablespoon chopped fresh dill
- 1/2 teaspoon dried thyme
- Salt and freshly ground black pepper, to taste

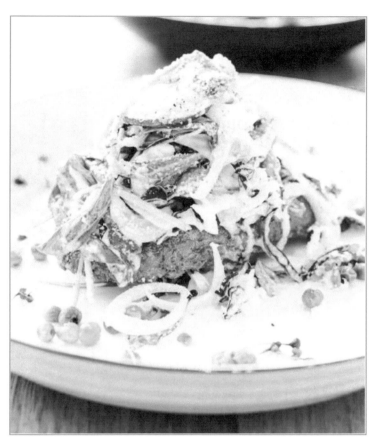

## Directions

1. In a large bowl, combine shredded chicken, grapes, celery, and red onion (if using).
2. In a small bowl, whisk together yogurt, lemon juice, dill, thyme, salt, and pepper.
3. Pour the dressing over the chicken salad and toss gently to coat..

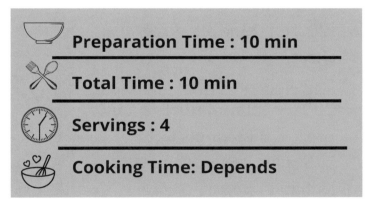

Preparation Time : 10 min

Total Time : 10 min

Servings : 4

Cooking Time: Depends

## Nutritional Information

- Calories: 220
- Fat: 3g
- Carbohydrates: 15g
- Sugar: 10g
- Protein: 25g

## Ingredients

- 2 skinless salmon fillets (4-6 ounces each)
- 1 lemon, thinly sliced
- 1 tablespoon fresh dill, chopped
- Salt and freshly ground black pepper, to taste

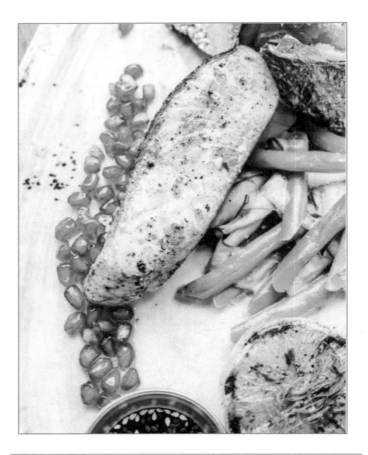

## Directions

1. Preheat oven to 400°F (200°C). Line a baking sheet with parchment paper.
2. Place salmon fillets on the prepared baking sheet. Season generously with salt and pepper.
3. Top each fillet with lemon slices and sprinkle with fresh dill.
4. Bake for 12-15 minutes, or until the salmon is cooked through and flakes easily with a fork.

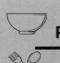 **Preparation Time : 5 min**

**Total Time : 10 min**

 **Servings : 2**

 **Cooking Time: 20 min**

## Nutritional Information

- Calories: 220
- Fat: 12g
- Carbs: 0g
- Protein: 30g

## Ingredients

- 1/2 cup non-fat Greek yogurt
- 1 tablespoon lemon juice
- 1 tablespoon olive oil
- 2 cloves garlic, minced
- 1 teaspoon dried oregano
- 1/2 teaspoon ground cumin
- 1/4 teaspoon smoked paprika
- 1/4 teaspoon salt
- 1/8 teaspoon black pepper
- 1 pound boneless, skinless chicken breasts or thighs

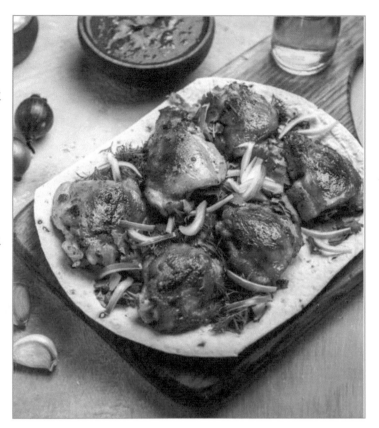

## Directions

1. In a large bowl, whisk together yogurt, lemon juice, olive oil, garlic, oregano, cumin, paprika, salt, and pepper. Add chicken and toss to coat. Cover and refrigerate for at least 30 minutes, or up to 4 hours for deeper flavor.
2. Preheat grill or grill pan to medium heat. Grill chicken for 5-7 minutes per side, or until cooked through. An internal temperature of 165°F is ideal.

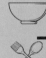 **Preparation Time : 5 min**

 **Total Time : 10 min**

 **Servings : 4**

 **Cooking Time: 20 min**

## Nutritional Information

- Calories: 200
- Protein: 30g
- Fat: 5g
- Carbs: 0g

## Ingredients

- 2 cups shredded cooked chicken breast
- ½ cup buffalo sauce
- ¼ cup plain non-fat Greek yogurt
- 2 tablespoons light cream cheese, softened
- 1 teaspoon garlic powder
- ½ teaspoon onion powder
- ¼ teaspoon paprika
- Salt and pepper to taste
- 8 celery stalks, trimmed and halved crosswise
- Optional garnish: chopped fresh parsley or chives

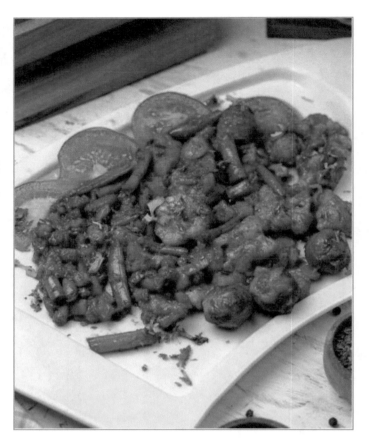

## Directions

1. In a mixing bowl, combine shredded chicken, buffalo sauce, Greek yogurt, cream cheese, garlic powder, onion powder, paprika, salt, and pepper. Mix until well combined.
2. Spoon the buffalo chicken mixture into the cavity of each celery stalk, distributing evenly.
3. Garnish with chopped fresh parsley or chives, if desired.
4. Serve immediately and enjoy the fiery bliss of Buffalo Chicken Celery Bites.

 **Preparation Time : 15 min**

 **Total Time : 10 min**

 **Servings : 4**

 **Cooking Time: 30 min**

## Nutritional Information

- Calories: 120 | Total Fat: 2g
- Saturated Fat: 0.5g | Cholesterol: 45mg
- Sodium: 590mg | Total Carbohydrates: 3g
- Dietary Fiber: 1g | Sugars: 1g
- Protein: 20g

# SNACKS AND APPETIZERS

Recipes

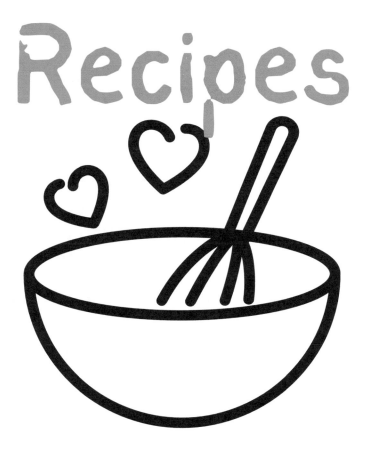

# EDAMAME

## Ingredients

- 2 cups frozen shelled edamame
- Water
- Pinch of sea salt (optional)

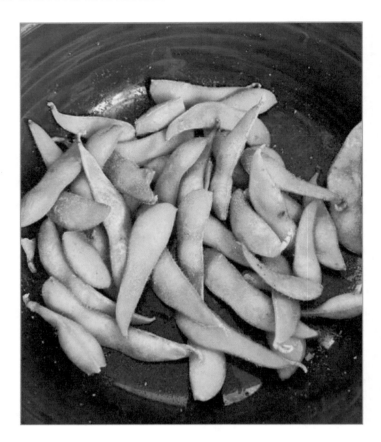

## Directions

1. In a saucepan, bring water to a boil. Add the edamame and cook for 3-5 minutes, or until tender-crisp.
2. Drain the edamame, discarding the water. Season with a pinch of sea salt, if desired.

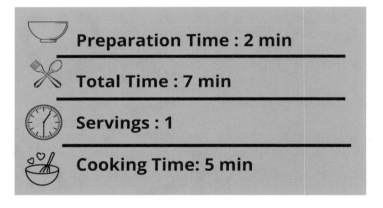

Preparation Time : 2 min

Total Time : 7 min

Servings : 1

Cooking Time: 5 min

## Nutritional Information

- Calories: 120
- Fat: 4.5g
- Carbohydrates: 11g
- Fiber: 5g
- Protein: 11g

# AIR-POPPED POPCORN

## Ingredients

- 1/3 cup Popcorn Kernels

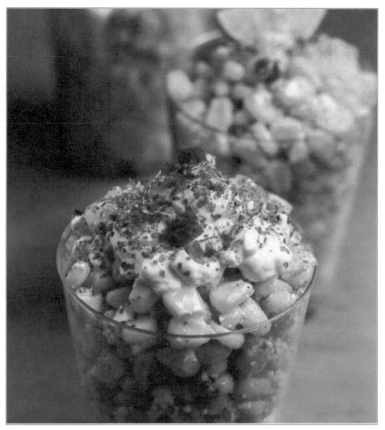

## Directions

1. Heat your air popper according to the manufacturer's instructions.
2. Add the popcorn kernels and turn on the popper.
3. Shake the popper occasionally to ensure even popping.
4. Once the popping slows to a few pops per minute, turn off the popper and transfer the popcorn to a large bowl.

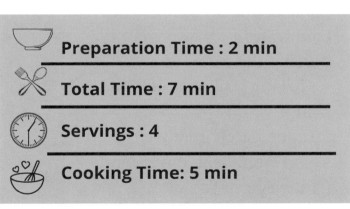

Preparation Time : 2 min

Total Time : 7 min

Servings : 4

Cooking Time: 5 min

## Nutritional Information

- Calories: 130 | Fat: 1g
- Saturated Fat: 0g | Cholesterol: 0mg
- Sodium: 1mg | Carbohydrates: 25g
- Fiber: 1g | Sugar: 1g
- Protein: 3g

# HARD-BOILED EGGS

## Ingredients

- 1 large, cold egg
- Water, to cover

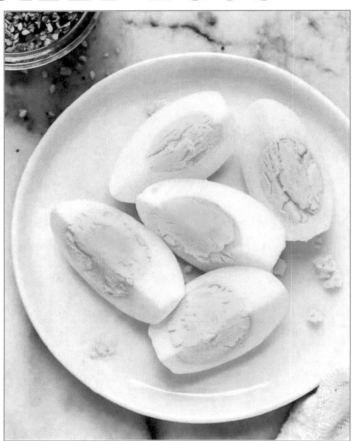

## Directions

1. Gently place the egg in a saucepan and cover with cold water.
2. Bring the water to a rolling boil over medium heat.
3. Immediately remove the pan from heat, cover, and let the egg sit for 12 minutes.
4. Drain the hot water and run cold water over the egg until cool enough to handle.
5. Peel and enjoy.

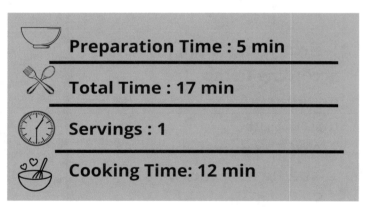

Preparation Time : 5 min

Total Time : 17 min

Servings : 1

Cooking Time: 12 min

## Nutritional Information

- Calories: 78 | Fat: 5g
- Saturated Fat: 1.5g | Cholesterol: 186mg
- Sodium: 61mg | Carbohydrates: 1g
- Protein: 6g

# PICKLES

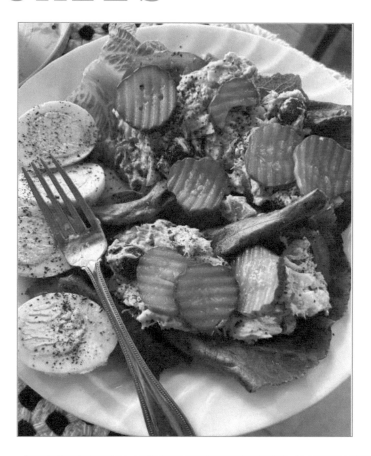

## Ingredients

- 1 Kirby cucumber, thinly sliced
- 1/2 cup distilled white vinegar
- 1/2 cup water
- 1 tablespoon pickling spice blend (available pre-mixed in most grocery stores)
- 1 garlic clove, smashed
- Fresh dill sprig (optional)

## Directions

1. In a clean, pint-sized mason jar, layer the cucumber slices.
2. In a small saucepan, combine vinegar, water, pickling spice, and garlic clove. Bring to a simmer, just until the spice releases its aroma.
3. Remove from heat and let cool slightly.
4. Pour the cooled pickling liquid over the cucumbers in the jar. Add the dill sprig, if using.
5. Seal the jar tightly and refrigerate for at least 12 hours, or up to 2 weeks for a more powerfully pickled flavor.

 **Preparation Time : 5 min**

 **Total Time : 5 min**

 **Servings : 2**

 **Cooking Time: N/A**

## Nutritional Information

- Calories: 5
- Fat: 0g
- Carbohydrates: 1g
- Sugar: 0g
- Sodium: 180mg

# SOUP BROTH

## Ingredients

- 1 tablespoon olive oil
- 1 medium onion, chopped
- 2 carrots, chopped
- 2 celery stalks, chopped
- 2 cloves garlic, minced
- 1 teaspoon dried thyme
- 1 teaspoon dried rosemary
- 8 cups low-sodium chicken broth (or vegetable broth for a vegan option)
- 1 bay leaf
- Freshly ground black pepper, to taste

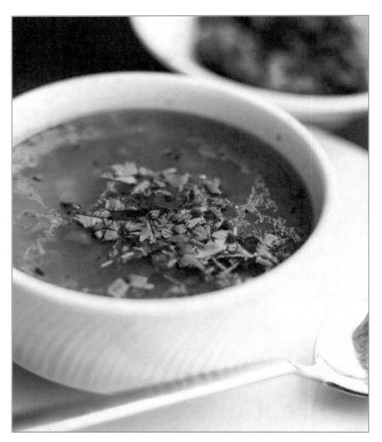

## Directions

1. Heat olive oil in a large pot over medium heat. Add onion, carrots, and celery. Sauté for 5 minutes, until softened.
2. Stir in garlic, thyme, and rosemary. Cook for 1 minute more.
3. Pour in chicken broth and add the bay leaf. Season with pepper.
4. Bring to a boil, then reduce heat and simmer for 40 minutes.
5. Strain the broth, discarding the solids.

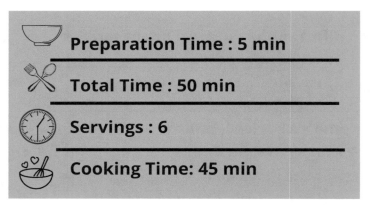

Preparation Time : 5 min

Total Time : 50 min

Servings : 6

Cooking Time: 45 min

## Nutritional Information

- Calories: 20
- Fat: 1g
- Carbohydrates: 2g
- Sugar: 1g
- Protein: 2g

# ROASTED CHICKPEAS

## Ingredients

- 1 can (15 oz) chickpeas, drained and rinsed
- 1 tablespoon olive oil spray (0 Points)
- 1 teaspoon garlic powder
- 1/2 teaspoon smoked paprika
- 1/4 teaspoon cayenne pepper (optional, for a kick)
- Salt and freshly ground black pepper, to taste

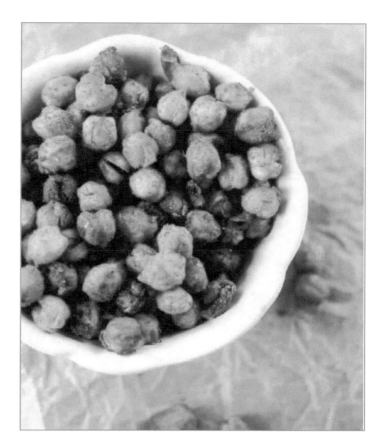

## Directions

1. Preheat your oven to 400°F (200°C). Lightly coat a baking sheet with olive oil spray.
2. In a bowl, toss the chickpeas with garlic powder, paprika, cayenne pepper (if using), salt, and pepper. Spread the seasoned chickpeas on the prepared baking sheet in a single layer.
3. Roast for 45-50 minutes, shaking the pan occasionally, until the chickpeas are golden brown and crispy. Let cool slightly before serving.

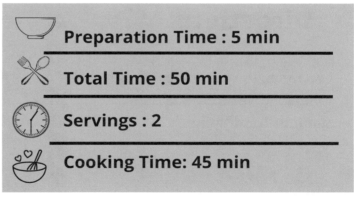

Preparation Time : 5 min

Total Time : 50 min

Servings : 2

Cooking Time: 45 min

## Nutritional Information

- Calories: 160 | Fat: 6g
- Saturated Fat: 1g | Cholesterol: 0mg
- Sodium: 80mg (depending on added salt)
- Carbohydrates: 20g | Fiber: 6g
- Sugar: 4g | Protein: 8g

# CUCUMBER SLICES WITH HUMMUS

## Ingredients

- 1 large cucumber, thinly sliced
- 1/2 cup hummus

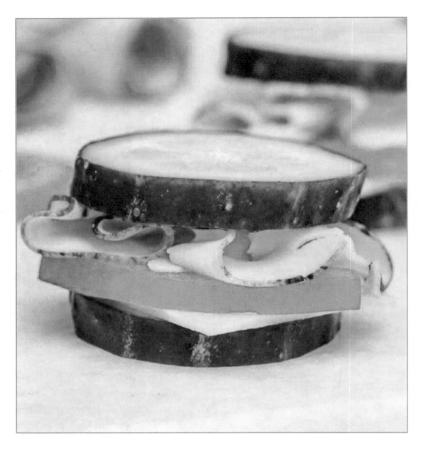

## Directions

1. Arrange the cucumber slices on a plate. Serve alongside the hummus for dipping.

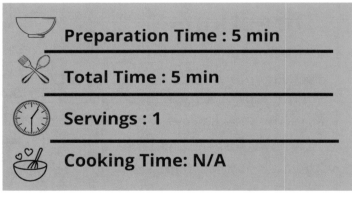

| | |
|---|---|
| 🍽 | **Preparation Time : 5 min** |
| 🍴 | **Total Time : 5 min** |
| 🕐 | **Servings : 1** |
| 🥣 | **Cooking Time: N/A** |

## Nutritional Information

- Calories: 30
- Fat: 0g
- Carbs: 6g
- Fiber: 1g
- Sugar: 2g
- Protein: 1g

# APPLE SLICES WITH ALMOND BUTTER

## Ingredients

- 1 large apple, thinly sliced
- 2 tablespoons almond butter

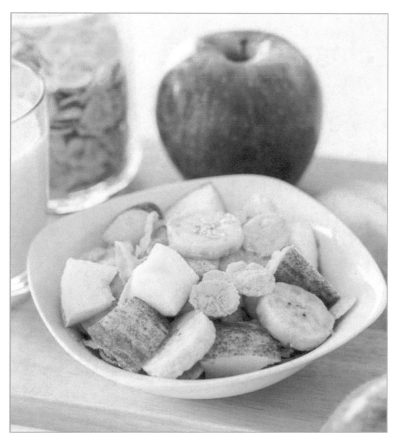

## Directions

1. Arrange apple slices on a plate.
2. Top with almond butter for dipping.

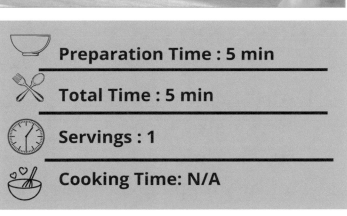

| | |
|---|---|
| 🥣 | **Preparation Time : 5 min** |
| 🍴 | **Total Time : 5 min** |
| 🕐 | **Servings : 1** |
| 🥣 | **Cooking Time: N/A** |

## Nutritional Information

- Calories: 190
- Fat: 9g
- Carbs: 25g
- Fiber: 4g
- Sugar: 19g
- Protein: 4g

## Ingredients

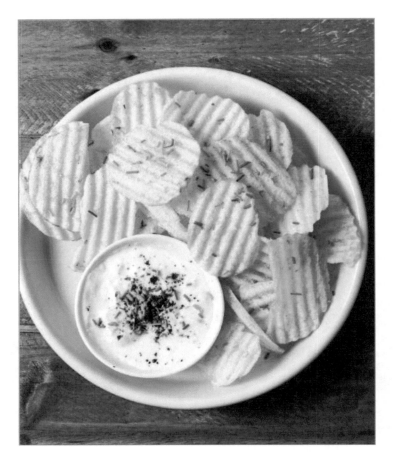

- 2 celery stalks, trimmed and cut into bite-sized sticks
- 2 tablespoons Neufchâtel cheese, softened

## Directions

1. Wash and trim the celery stalks, then cut them into sticks for easy dipping.
2. Serve the celery sticks alongside the softened Neufchâtel cheese for a delightful 0-point snack.

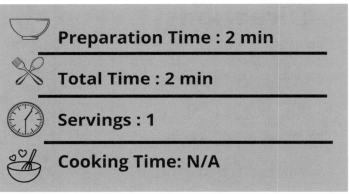

| | |
|---|---|
| Preparation Time : 2 min | |
| Total Time : 2 min | |
| Servings : 1 | |
| Cooking Time: N/A | |

## Nutritional Information

- Calories: 70
- Fat: 3.5g
- Carbohydrates: 5g
- Fiber: 2g
- Sugar: 1g
- Protein: 2g

# DESSERTS

## Recipes

# SUGAR-FREE JELLO CUPS

## Ingredients

- 1 (3 oz.) package sugar-free flavored gelatin
- 1 cup boiling water
- 1 cup unsweetened flavored sparkling water (optional, for extra fizz)
- Fresh fruit (optional, for garnish)

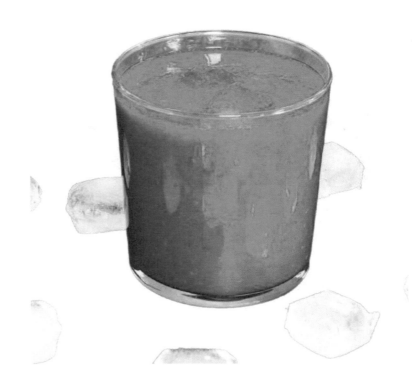

## Directions

1. In a heatproof bowl, whisk together the gelatin powder and boiling water until the powder dissolves completely.
2. Stir in the sparkling water (if using) and pour the mixture into individual serving cups.
3. (Optional) Gently stir in fresh fruit for a pop of color and texture.
4. Refrigerate for at least 4 hours, or until set.

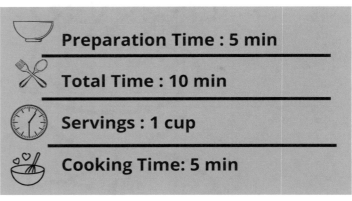

Preparation Time : 5 min

Total Time : 10 min

Servings : 1 cup

Cooking Time: 5 min

## Nutritional Information

- Calories: 5
- Fat: 0g
- Carbohydrates: 1g
- Sugar: 0g
- Protein: 1g

# FRUIT KABOBS

## Ingredients

- 1 cup fresh strawberries, hulled and halved
- 1 cup blueberries
- 1 medium kiwi, peeled and sliced
- 1 medium cantaloupe, peeled and cubed
- 1 honeydew melon, peeled and cubed
- 1 mango, peeled and cubed (optional)
- 1 cup raspberries (optional)
- Wooden skewers (soaked in water for 10 minutes to prevent burning)

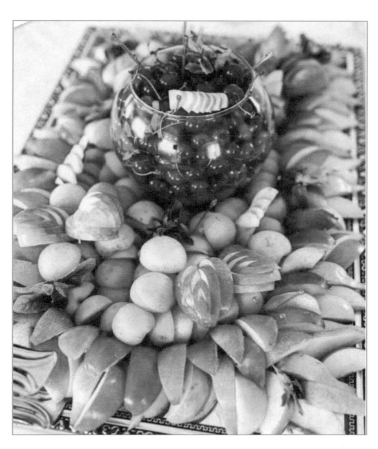

## Directions

1.Assemble the kabobs: Thread the fruits alternately onto skewers, creating a vibrant rainbow pattern.

 **Preparation Time : 10 min**

 **Total Time : 10 min**

 **Servings : 4**

 **Cooking Time: N/A**

## Nutritional Information

- Calories: 60
- Fat: 0g
- Carbohydrates: 15g
- Sugar: 10g
- Protein: 1g

# CHIA SEED PUDDING

## Ingredients

- 2 tablespoons chia seeds
- 1 cup unsweetened almond milk (or other zero-point milk of your choice)
- ½ teaspoon vanilla extract (optional)
- Fresh berries or a sprinkle of cinnamon for topping (optional)

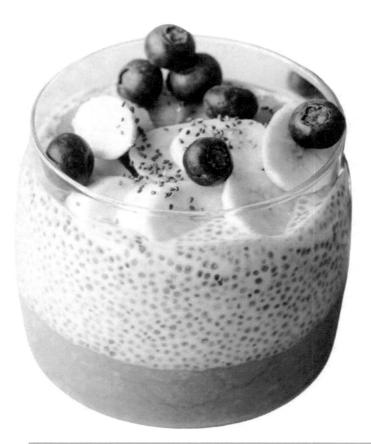

## Directions

1. In a jar or container, whisk together chia seeds, almond milk, and vanilla extract (if using).
2. Stir well, ensuring there are no dry pockets of chia seeds.
3. Refrigerate for at least 2 hours, or preferably overnight, to allow the chia seeds to absorb the liquid and thicken into a pudding consistency.
4. When ready to serve, stir the pudding and top with fresh berries or a sprinkle of cinnamon, if desired.

 **Preparation Time : 5 min**

 **Total Time : 5 min**

 **Servings : 1**

 **Cooking Time: N/A**

## Nutritional Information

- Calories: 138
- Fat: 8g
- Carbohydrates: 11g
- Fiber: 5g
- Protein: 4g

# CUCUMBER MINT SORBET

## Ingredients

- 1 large seedless cucumber, peeled and chopped
- 1/2 cup packed fresh mint leaves
- 1/4 cup lime juice (freshly squeezed for best flavor)
- 2 tablespoons water

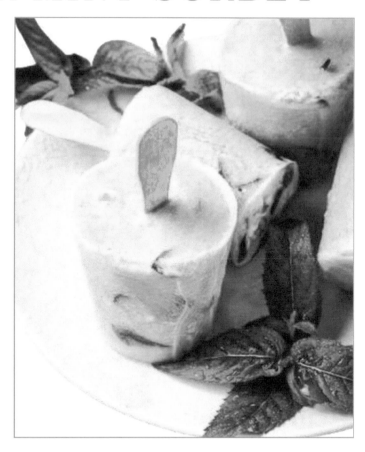

## Directions

1. Combine all ingredients in a high-powered blender and blend until smooth and creamy.
2. Pour the mixture into a shallow freezer-safe container and freeze for at least 4 hours, or until completely solid.
3. Remove from the freezer and let sit for 5-10 minutes to soften slightly before scooping.

 **Preparation Time : 5 min**

 **Total Time : 5 min**

 **Servings : 1**

 **Cooking Time: N/A**

## Nutritional Information

- Calories: 40
- Fat: 0g
- Carbohydrates: 10g
- Fiber: 1g
- Sugar: 8g
- Protein: 1g

## Ingredients

- 1 round rice cake
- 1 tablespoon almond butter

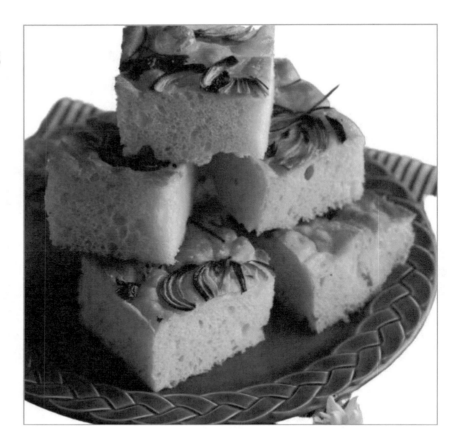

## Directions

1. Spread the almond butter over the rice cake. Savor the delightful combination.

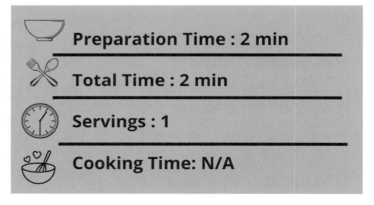

**Preparation Time : 2 min**

**Total Time : 2 min**

**Servings : 1**

**Cooking Time: N/A**

## Nutritional Information

- Calories: 115
- Fat: 8g
- Carbs: 18g
- Fiber: 2g
- Sugar: 1g
- Protein: 3g

# STUFFED DATES

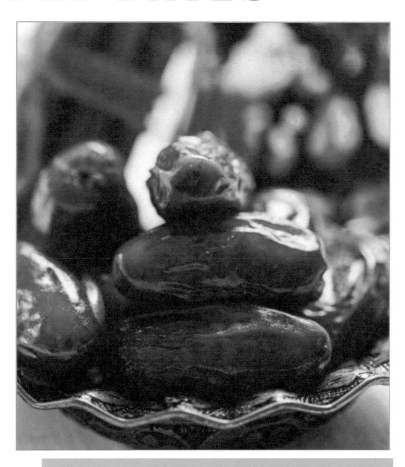

## Ingredients

- 12 Medjool Dates (or Deglet Noor)
- ½ cup Almonds, roughly chopped
- ½ cup Ricotta Cheese
- 1 tablespoon Honey
- ½ teaspoon Orange Zest
- Pinch of Ground Cinnamon

## Directions

1. With a sharp knife, make a small slit along the side of each date and remove the pit.
2. In a small bowl, combine the ricotta cheese, honey, orange zest, and cinnamon.
3. Using a teaspoon, gently stuff the ricotta mixture into each date cavity.
4. Press an almond half or sliver onto the top of each stuffed date.

 **Preparation Time : 5 min**

 **Total Time : 5 min**

 **Servings : 6**

 **Cooking Time: N/A**

## Nutritional Information

- Calories: 180
- Fat: 8g
- Carbohydrates: 23g
- Fiber: 3g
- Sugar: 18g
- Protein: 2g

# MIXED BERRY SMOOTHIE

## Ingredients

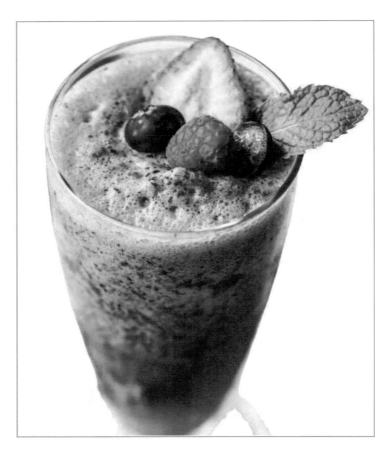

- 1 cup frozen mixed berries (strawberries, blueberries, raspberries)
- ½ banana, frozen
- ¾ cup unsweetened almond milk (or water)
- ½ cup plain, fat-free Greek yogurt

## Directions

1. Combine all ingredients in a blender and blend until smooth and creamy.
2. Pour into a glass and enjoy the delightful melody of flavors.

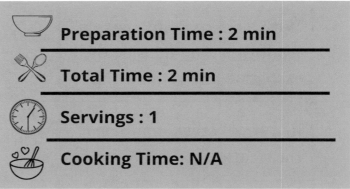

Preparation Time : 2 min

Total Time : 2 min

Servings : 1

Cooking Time: N/A

## Nutritional Information

- Calories: 180
- Fat: 3g
- Carbohydrates: 28g
- Fiber: 4g
- Sugar: 15g (naturally occurring sugars)
- Protein: 10g

# BANANA ICE CREAM

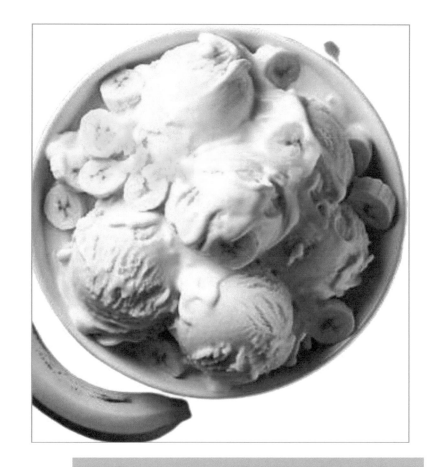

## Ingredients

- 2 ripe bananas, peeled and chopped

## Directions

1. Place the chopped bananas in a freezer-safe container or bag. Seal tightly and banish them to the frozen tundra for at least 2 hours, or ideally overnight. The riper the bananas, the sweeter the "ice cream" will be.

2. Retrieve your frozen banana shards and add them to a high-powered blender or food processor. Blend until smooth and impossibly creamy, scraping down the sides as needed.

 **Preparation Time : 5 min**

 **Total Time : 5 min**

 **Servings : 1**

 **Cooking Time: N/A**

## Nutritional Information

- Calories: 105
- Fat: 0.5g
- Carbohydrates: 27g
- Fiber: 3g
- Sugar: 14g
- Protein: 1g

## Ingredients

- 1 cup plain Greek yogurt (0% fat)
- 1 tablespoon honey
- 1/2 teaspoon ground cinnamon

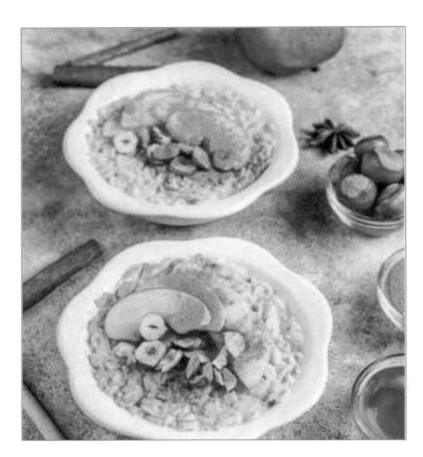

## Directions

1. In a small bowl, combine the Greek yogurt, honey, and cinnamon. Stir well to combine.

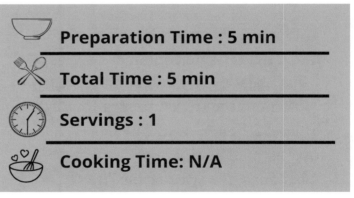

Preparation Time : 5 min

Total Time : 5 min

Servings : 1

Cooking Time: N/A

## Nutritional Information

- Calories: 105
- Fat: 0.5g
- Carbohydrates: 27g
- Fiber: 3g
- Sugar: 14g
- Protein: 1g

# WATERMELON POPSICLES

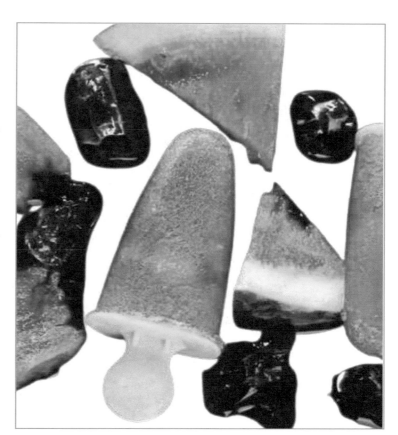

## Ingredients

- 4 cups cubed seedless watermelon
- 1/2 cup fresh lime juice
- 2 tablespoons honey (optional)
- 1/4 cup fresh mint leaves, chopped
- 6 popsicle molds
- 6 popsicle sticks

## Directions

1. Blend watermelon, lime juice, and honey until smooth.
2. Stir in chopped mint leaves.
3. Pour mixture into popsicle molds.
4. Insert popsicle sticks and freeze for at least 4 hours or until solid.
5. Remove from molds and enjoy!

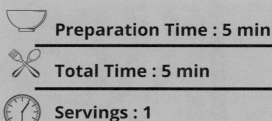

**Preparation Time : 5 min**

**Total Time : 5 min**

**Servings : 1**

**Cooking Time: N/A**

## Nutritional Information

- Calories: 105
- Fat: 0.5g
- Carbohydrates: 27g
- Fiber: 3g
- Sugar: 14g
- Protein: 1g

# MAIN COURSE
## Recipes

# BAKED SALMON WITH DILL

## Ingredients

- 1 (4-ounce) skinless salmon fillet
- 1 tablespoon fresh dill, chopped
- 1 tablespoon freshly squeezed lemon juice
- Salt and freshly ground black pepper, to taste

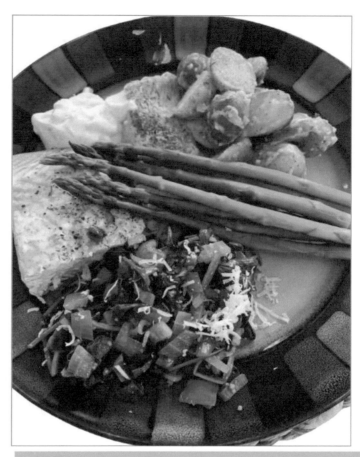

## Directions

1. Preheat oven to 400°F (200°C). Line a baking sheet with parchment paper.
2. Place the salmon fillet on the prepared baking sheet. Season generously with salt and pepper.
3. Sprinkle the chopped dill over the salmon and drizzle with lemon juice.
4. Bake for 12-15 minutes, or until the salmon flakes easily with a fork.

 **Preparation Time : 5 min**

 **Total Time : 20 min**

 **Servings : 1**

 **Cooking Time: 15 min**

## Nutritional Information

- Calories: 170
- Protein: 22g
- Fat: 7g
- Carbs: 0g
- pen_spark

# EGGPLANT PARMESAN

## Ingredients

- 1 medium eggplant (about 1 pound)
- Salt
- 2 large egg whites, lightly beaten
- 1/2 cup fat-free ricotta cheese
- 1/4 cup shredded part-skim mozzarella cheese
- 1 tablespoon grated Parmesan cheese
- 1 (14.5-ounce) can diced tomatoes, undrained
- 1 tablespoon chopped fresh basil, or 1 teaspoon dried basil
  Freshly ground black pepper, to taste
- Cooking spray

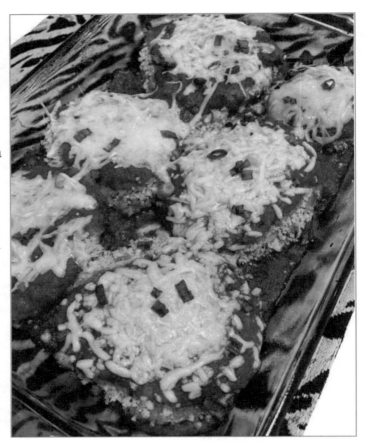

## Directions

1. Preheat oven to 400°F (200°C). Slice eggplant into 1/2-inch rounds. Arrange on a baking sheet, sprinkle with salt, and let sit for 10 minutes. Pat dry with paper towels.
2. Dip eggplant slices in egg whites, then coat with cooking spray. Bake for 20-25 minutes, flipping halfway through, until golden brown and tender.
3. While eggplant bakes, combine ricotta cheese, mozzarella cheese, Parmesan cheese, diced tomatoes, and basil in a bowl. Season with black pepper.
4. Spread a thin layer of sauce in a baking dish. Top with half of the eggplant slices, followed by half of the remaining sauce. Repeat with remaining eggplant and sauce.
5. Bake for 10-15 minutes, or until heated through and cheese is melted.

 **Preparation Time : 15 min**

 **Total Time : 50 min**

 **Servings : 4**

 **Cooking Time: 35 min**

## Nutritional Information

- Calories: 170 | Fat: 4g
- Saturated Fat: 1g | Cholesterol: 10mg
- Sodium: 320mg | Carbohydrates: 22g
- Fiber: 4g | Sugar: 8g
- Protein: 12g

## Ingredients

- 1 cup shelled edamame, frozen or fresh
- 1 tablespoon olive oil
- 1/4 teaspoon red pepper flakes (adjust to your spice preference)
- 1/4 teaspoon garlic powder
- Salt and freshly ground black pepper, to taste
- 1 tablespoon chopped fresh parsley
- 1 tablespoon chopped fresh cilantro

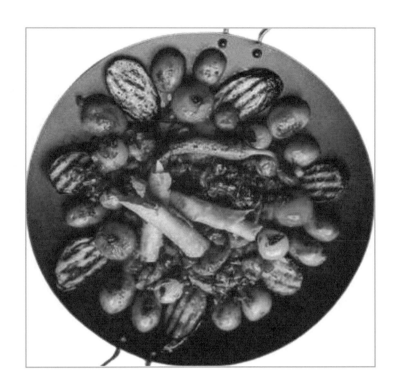

## Directions

1. If using frozen edamame, cook according to package instructions. Drain and pat dry.
2. Heat olive oil in a large skillet over medium heat. Add edamame, red pepper flakes, and garlic powder. Cook for 3-4 minutes, stirring occasionally, until edamame is heated through and slightly blistered.
3. Season with salt and pepper to taste. Remove from heat and stir in parsley and cilantro.

 **Preparation Time : 5 min**

 **Total Time : 10 min**

 **Servings : 2**

 **Cooking Time: 5 min**

## Nutritional Information

- Calories: 120
- Fat: 6g
- Carbohydrates: 10g
- Fiber: 5g
- Protein: 8g

## Ingredients

- 4 oz (113g) uncooked whole wheat or zero-point pasta (like chickpea pasta)
- ½ lb (225g) raw, peeled, and deveined shrimp
- 1 tablespoon olive oil
- 2 cloves garlic, minced
- ½ teaspoon dried oregano
- ¼ teaspoon red pepper flakes (optional)
- Juice of 1 lemon
- ¼ cup chopped fresh parsley
- Salt and freshly ground black pepper, to taste

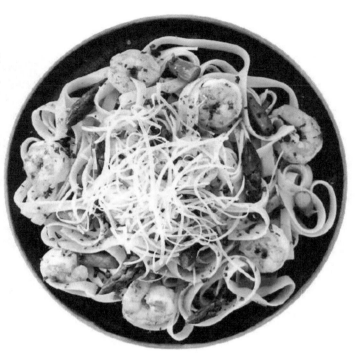

## Directions

1. Cook the pasta according to package directions, reserving 1/4 cup of the pasta water before draining.
2. While the pasta boils, heat olive oil in a large skillet over medium heat. Add shrimp and cook for 2-3 minutes per side, or until pink and opaque. Remove shrimp from the pan and set aside.
3. Add garlic to the pan and cook for 30 seconds, until fragrant. Stir in lemon juice, reserved pasta water, and salt and pepper.
4. Add cooked pasta and shrimp back to the pan, tossing to coat with the sauce. Garnish with fresh parsley and serve immediately.

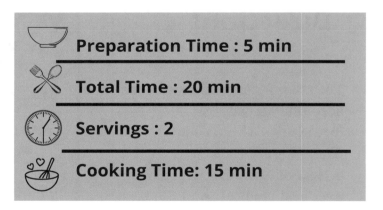

**Preparation Time : 5 min**

**Total Time : 20 min**

**Servings : 2**

**Cooking Time: 15 min**

## Nutritional Information

- Calories: 380
- Fat: 12g
- Carbohydrates: 38g
- Fiber: 4g
- Protein: 28g

## Ingredients

- 2 large eggs
- ½ teaspoon olive oil
- ½ cup chopped red or yellow bell pepper
- ½ cup chopped mushrooms
- ½ cup chopped baby spinach
- Pinch of salt
- Pinch of black pepper

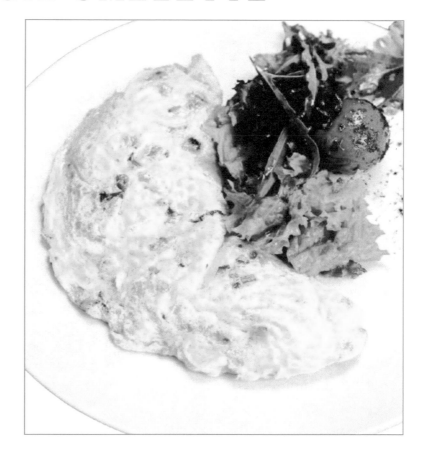

## Directions

1. In a small bowl, whisk together the eggs with a pinch of salt and pepper.
2. Heat olive oil in a non-stick pan over medium heat. Add the bell pepper and mushrooms, and cook until softened, about 3 minutes.
3. Push the vegetables to one side of the pan. Pour in the egg mixture, tilting the pan to spread evenly.
4. As the eggs begin to set, sprinkle the spinach over the omelette. Let cook until the bottom is golden brown and the top is mostly set.
5. Fold the omelette in half and serve immediately.

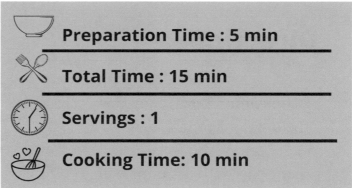

Preparation Time : 5 min

Total Time : 15 min

Servings : 1

Cooking Time: 10 min

## Nutritional Information

- Calories: 140
- Fat: 7g
- Carbohydrates: 2g
- Protein: 12g

# TUNA SALAD LETTUCE WRAPS

## Ingredients

- 1 (5-ounce) can chunk light tuna in water, drained
- 1/4 cup low-fat mayonnaise
- 1 tablespoon chopped red onion
- 1 tablespoon chopped celery
- 1/2 teaspoon dried dill weed
- 1/4 teaspoon black pepper
- 1 head romaine lettuce, leaves separated and washed

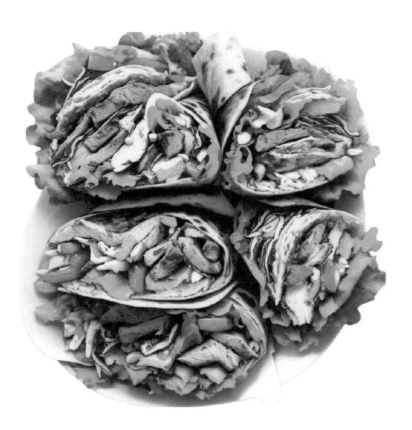

## Directions

1. In a medium bowl, combine the tuna, mayonnaise, red onion, celery, dill weed, and black pepper. Toss until well combined.
2. Fill each romaine lettuce leaf with a generous spoonful of the tuna salad mixture. Serve immediately.

 **Preparation Time : 5 min**

 **Total Time : 5 min**

 **Servings : 4**

 **Cooking Time: N/A**

## Nutritional Information

- Calories: 170
- Fat: 5g
- Carbohydrates: 5g
- Fiber: 1g
- Protein: 20g

# GRILLED VEGETABLE SALAD

## Ingredients

- 1 red bell pepper, sliced into thick strips
- 1 yellow bell pepper, sliced into thick strips
- 1 zucchini, sliced into thick rounds
- 1 red onion, cut into wedges
- 1 bunch asparagus, trimmed
- 2 tablespoons olive oil
- 1 tablespoon balsamic vinegar
- 1/2 teaspoon dried oregano
- 1/4 teaspoon smoked paprika
- Salt and freshly ground black pepper, to taste

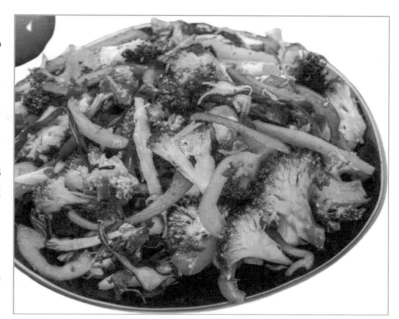

## Directions

1. In a large bowl, combine olive oil, balsamic vinegar, oregano, smoked paprika, salt, and pepper. Toss the vegetables to coat them evenly.
2. Preheat your grill to medium-high heat. Alternatively, preheat a grill pan over medium heat.
3. Grill the vegetables for 5-7 minutes per side, or until tender-crisp and slightly charred.

 **Preparation Time : 10 min**

 **Total Time : 30 min**

 **Servings : 4**

 **Cooking Time: 20 min**

## Nutritional Information

- Calories: 100
- Fat: 5g
- Carbohydrates: 10g
- Fiber: 3g
- Sugar: 5g
- Protein: 2g

## Ingredients

- 1 pound ground turkey breast (99% fat-free)
- 1 medium onion, chopped
- 1 green pepper, chopped (optional)
- 2 cloves garlic, minced
- 1 (15 oz) can diced tomatoes with green chilies, undrained
- 1 (15 oz) can black beans, rinsed and drained
- 1 (15 oz) can kidney beans, rinsed and drained
- 1 (15 oz) can corn, drained
- 1 (14.5 oz) can crushed tomatoes
- 2 tablespoons chili powder
- 1 tablespoon ground cumin
- 1 teaspoon dried oregano
- 1/2 teaspoon salt
- 1/4 teaspoon black pepper
-

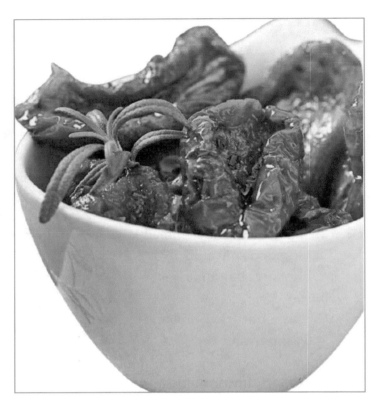

## Directions

1. In a large skillet, brown the ground turkey over medium heat. Drain any excess grease.
2. In your slow cooker, combine browned turkey, onion, green pepper (if using), garlic, diced tomatoes, black beans, kidney beans, corn, crushed tomatoes, chili powder, cumin, oregano, salt, and pepper. Stir well.
3. Cover and cook on low for 4 hours, or on high for 6 hours.

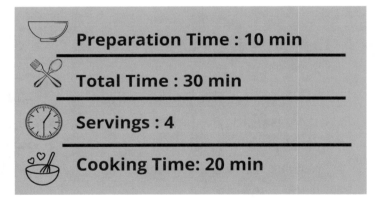

Preparation Time : 10 min

Total Time : 30 min

Servings : 4

Cooking Time: 20 min

## Nutritional Information

- Calories: 300
- Fat: 5g
- Carbohydrates: 30g
- Fiber: 10g
- Protein: 25g

# 30 DAYS
## Meal Plan

## DAY 1

- Breakfast: Fresh Fruit Salad
- Lunch: Turkey Taco Pasta Salad
- Dinner: Grilled Vegetable Salad

## DAY 2

- Breakfast: Apple and Cinnamon Barley Porridge
- Lunch: Lentil Soup
- Dinner: Lemon Garlic Shrimp Pasta

## DAY 3

- Breakfast: Tofu Scramble
- Lunch: Greek Chicken Salad
- Dinner: Veggie Omelette

## DAY 4

- Breakfast: Shakshuka
- Lunch: Buffalo Chicken Tostadas
- Dinner: Turkey Chili

## DAY 5

- Breakfast: Turkey Breakfast Sausage Patties
- Lunch: Chicken Taco Soup
- Dinner: Eggplant Parmesan

## DAY 6

- Breakfast: Muffin Tin Eggs
- Lunch: Black Bean Burgers
- Dinner: Baked Salmon with Lemon and Dill

---

## DAY 7

- Breakfast: Banana Berry Parfait
- Lunch: Chicken Bacon Tostadas
- Dinner: Grilled Portobello Mushrooms

---

## DAY 8

- Breakfast: Silverbeet and Dukkah Baked Eggs
- Lunch: Salmon with Roasted Vegetables
- Dinner: Veggie Omelette

---

## DAY 9

- BrBreakfast: Poached Eggs and Toast
- Lunch: Buffalo Chicken Celery Bites
- Dinner: Turkey Burgers

---

## DAY 10

- Breakfast: Bacon, Egg, and Spinach Bakes
- Lunch: Edamame
- Dinner: Lemon Garlic Shrimp Pasta

## DAY 11

- Breakfast: Poached Egg with Tomato Salsa
- Lunch: Chicken Taco Cupcakes
- Dinner: Eggplant Parmesan

## DAY 12

- Breakfast: Grilled Fruit Salad Bowl
- Lunch: Soup Broth
- Dinner: Greek Chicken Salad

## DAY 13

- Breakfast: Sweet Potato Breakfast Hash
- Lunch: Roasted Chickpeas
- Dinner: Buffalo Chicken Tostadas

## DAY 14

- Breakfast: Strawberry Oatmeal
- Lunch: Cucumber Slices with Hummus
- Dinner: Baked Salmon with Dill

## DAY 15

- Breakfast: Berry Baked Oats
- Lunch: Air-Popped Popcorn
- Dinner: Veggie Omelette

## DAY 16

- Breakfast: Pineapple Chicken and Rice Wraps
- Lunch: Turkey Taco Pasta Salad
- Dinner: Grilled Portobello Mushrooms

## DAY 17

- Breakfast: Buffalo Chicken Celery Bites
- Lunch: Lentil Soup
- Dinner: Lemon Garlic Shrimp Pasta

## DAY 18

- Breakfast: Yogurt Chicken Salad with Dressing
- Lunch: Soup Broth
- Dinner: Turkey Burgers

## DAY 19

- Breakfast: Baked Salmon with Lemon and Dill
- Lunch: Greek Yogurt with Honey and Cinnamon
- Dinner: Eggplant Parmesan

## DAY 20

- Breakfast: Buffalo Chicken Tostadas
- Lunch: Cucumber Slices with Hummus
- Dinner: Grilled Vegetable Salad

## DAY 21

- Breakfast: Strawberry Oatmeal
- Lunch: Roasted Chickpeas
- Dinner: Turkey Chili

## DAY 22

- Breakfast: Banana "Ice Cream"
- Lunch: Chicken Taco Cupcakes
- Dinner: Baked Salmon with Dill

## DAY 23

- Breakfast: Mixed Berry Smoothie
- Lunch: Tuna Salad Lettuce Wraps
- Dinner: Veggie Omelette

## DAY 24

- Breakfast: Chia Seed Pudding
- Lunch: Buffalo Chicken Celery Bites
- Dinner: Lemon Garlic Shrimp Pasta

## DAY 25

- Breakfast: Rice Cake with Almond Butter
- Lunch: Soup Broth
- Dinner: Turkey Burgers

## DAY 26

- Breakfast: Stuffed Dates
- Lunch: Greek Chicken Salad
- Dinner: Grilled Portobello Mushrooms

---

## DAY 27

- Breakfast: Greek Yogurt with Honey and Cinnamon
- Lunch: Edamame
- Dinner: Eggplant Parmesan

---

## DAY 28

- Breakfast: Watermelon Popsicles
- Lunch: Turkey Taco Pasta Salad
- Dinner: Lemon Garlic Shrimp Pasta

---

## DAY 29

- Breakfast: Greek Yogurt with Honey and Cinnamon
- Lunch: Lentil Soup
- Dinner: Grilled Vegetable Salad

---

## DAY 30

- Breakfast: Veggie Omelette
- Lunch: Chicken Taco Soup
- Dinner: Baked Salmon with Lemon and Dill

# CONCLUSION

You've started on a wonderful path of healthy change. With this cookbook as your guide, you've unlocked a world of delectable, zero-point meals that fuel your body while also satisfying your taste buds. Remember that weight loss is a marathon, not a sprint. Accept the process, appreciate your accomplishments, and, most importantly, enjoy the delicious food that supports your healthy lifestyle. Congratulations on taking responsibility of your health, and here's to a future full of rich tastes and long- term weight loss.

Made in United States
Troutdale, OR
06/29/2024

20892701R00046